Preggatinis™

Preggatinis™

Mixology for the Mom-to-Be

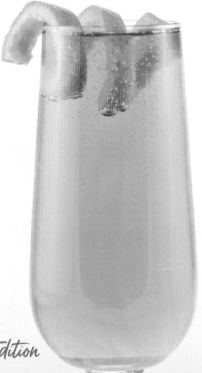

Second Edition

Natalie Bovis
The Liquid Muse

Photographs by
Claire Barrett

Globe
Pequot
Essex, Connecticut

Globe
Pequot

An imprint of Globe Pequot, the trade division of The Rowman & Littlefield
Publishing Group, Inc.
4501 Forbes Blvd., Ste. 200
Lanham, MD 20706
www.rowman.com

Distributed by NATIONAL BOOK NETWORK

British Library Cataloguing in Publication Information available

Library of Congress Cataloging-in-Publication Data

Names: Bovis-Nelsen, Natalie, author.
Title: Preggatinis : mixology for the mom-to-be / Natalie Bovis ;
    photographs by Claire Barrett.
Description: Second edition. | Essex, Connecticut : Globe Pequot, 2024. |
    Includes index.
Identifiers: LCCN 2023023678 (print) | LCCN 2023023679 (ebook) | ISBN
    9781493072620 (paper ; alk. paper) | ISBN 9781493072637 (electronic)
Subjects: LCSH: Non-alcoholic cocktails. | Pregnant women.
Classification: LCC TX815 .B745 2024 (print) | LCC TX815 (ebook) | DDC
    641.87/5—dc23/eng/20230519
LC record available at https://lccn.loc.gov/2023023678
LC ebook record available at https://lccn.loc.gov/2023023679

♾️™ The paper used in this publication meets the minimum requirements of
American National Standard for Information Sciences—Permanence of Paper for
Printed Library Materials, ANSI/NISO Z39.48-1992.

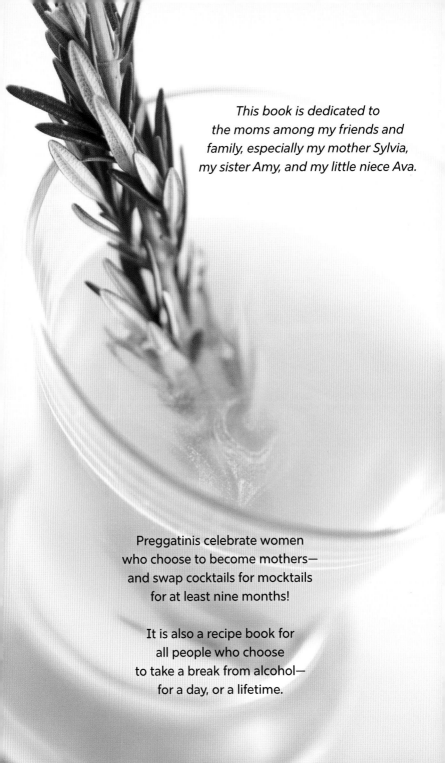

*This book is dedicated to
the moms among my friends and
family, especially my mother Sylvia,
my sister Amy, and my little niece Ava.*

Preggatinis celebrate women
who choose to become mothers—
and swap cocktails for mocktails
for at least nine months!

It is also a recipe book for
all people who choose
to take a break from alcohol—
for a day, or a lifetime.

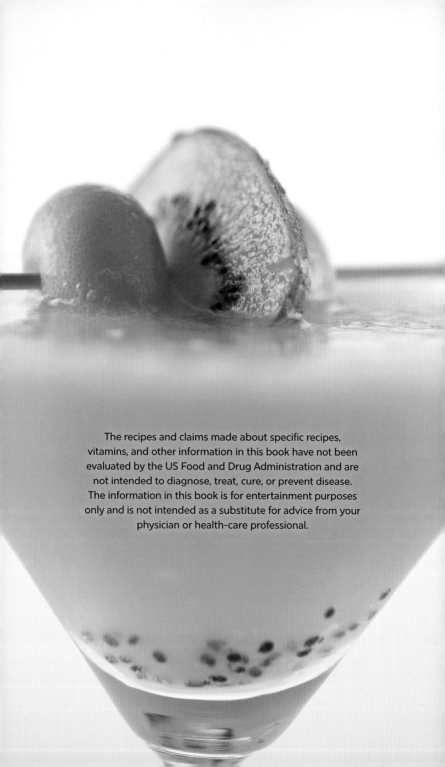

Every book is a labor of love and—like raising a child—it takes a village to get it done well.

Many thanks to Claire Barrett, whose gorgeous photos bring my recipes to life; Lilly Ghahremani, who has guided my book career for two decades; Mary Norris, who was my editor on the first round of *Preggatinis* in 2007; and the entire Globe Pequot team for helping make this new, updated version of *Preggatinis* happen in 2024.

Contents

Prelude to a Preggatini

Welcome to one of the biggest decisions of your life . . . to give up cocktails for nine months! Never fear, this home bartending guide keeps the fun and glamour of cocktail culture in mocktail mixing. Preggatinis are colorful, tasty, and healthful. Best of all, you'll be well equipped to "belly up" to your own Preggatini home bar.

Not to be confused with the goopy, syrupy, unappetizing mocktails you may have encountered in the past, a Preggatini is made with freshly squeezed fruit and vegetable juices, muddled herbs, and farmers' market quality produce. There are recipes for homemade syrups and shrubs that can be used for cocktails, too, along with "extra kick" suggestions for non-preggie pals. And the Preggatini Party chapter includes themed food and drink menus for the most delicious gender reveal or baby shower ever!

Preggatinis is the original nonalcoholic cocktail guide for sipping your way through this special time when you are the star, the VIP—when the world seems to revolve around your belly! Hold on to this book after baby's arrival because the recipes and tips will serve you well for years to come. Besides, you never know when you may reach for the Preggatini shaker again . . .

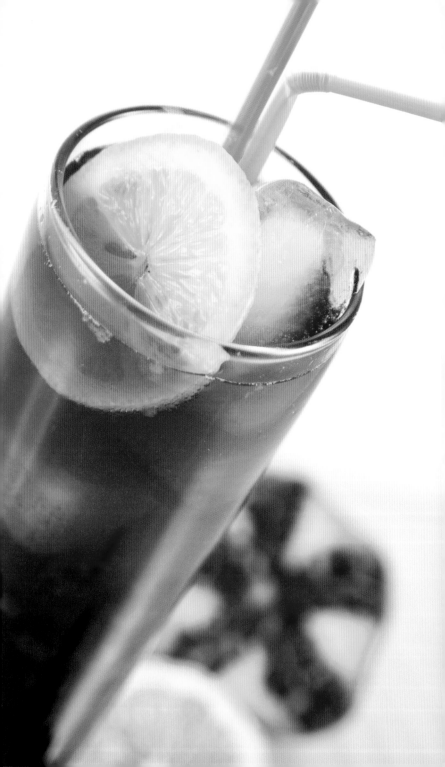

Part One
The Liquid Muse Home Bar Basics

————

The nursery is baby's nest, haven, safety zone. In the coming months you'll pick the perfect crib, changing table, and hanging mobile. You'll stock up on diapers, wet wipes, and onesies. You'll buy bottles, bags, and baby baubles. Baby's "happy place" will be ready and waiting. Meanwhile, you deserve your very own chill-out zone at your Preggatini Home Bar!

The Tools of the Trade

Can an artist paint without a brush? Can a guitarist strum a melody without an instrument? Can you shake and stir without a few basic bar tools? Well, actually, you can! I've included some household alternatives throughout this list of bartending gadgets. Whether or not you stock your Preggatini home bar with all the bells and whistles, you can still make great drinks like a pro.

BAR SPOON: This looks like a teaspoon with a very long stem, ideal for stirring ingredients in a tall glass. A household option would be a teaspoon or iced-tea spoon.

CITRUS PRESS: This is a handheld tool used to squeeze juice from lemons and limes. Simply cut the citrus in half, place the cut side down over the holes, and press. If you don't have one, simply squeeze by hand.

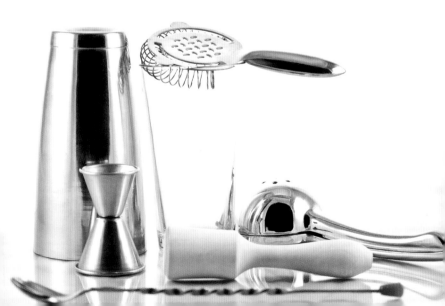

COCKTAIL SHAKER: There are many kinds of shakers, including three-piece shakers (a tin, a slotted lid and a little cap), Boston shakers (clear mixing glass with metal tin and Hawthorne strainer), and shaking tins (a big tin and a little one). Whichever you prefer will get the job done. A household option would be to put the ingredients and ice in a large mason jar, close the lid, and give it a good shake.

JIGGER: Used for measuring small amounts of liquid. These come in different sizes, and the large side of an hourglass-shaped jigger measures double the small side. A household option would be measuring spoons used for baking.

MUDDLER: This is basically a pestle with a longer handle so it can reach to the bottom of a mixing glass. "Muddle" by pressing the fruit, herbs, etc., in a downward, rotating motion to release their oils, juices, and flavors. If you don't have one, simply use the round part of a tablespoon or the handle of spatula to crush the ingredients.

PARING KNIFE AND CUTTING BOARD: You will need these for chopping, slicing, and peeling fresh produce.

STRAINER: If your shaker doesn't have a built-in strainer, a Hawthorne strainer has a coil to help hold back bits of fruit or herbs. A household option would be a small kitchen sieve.

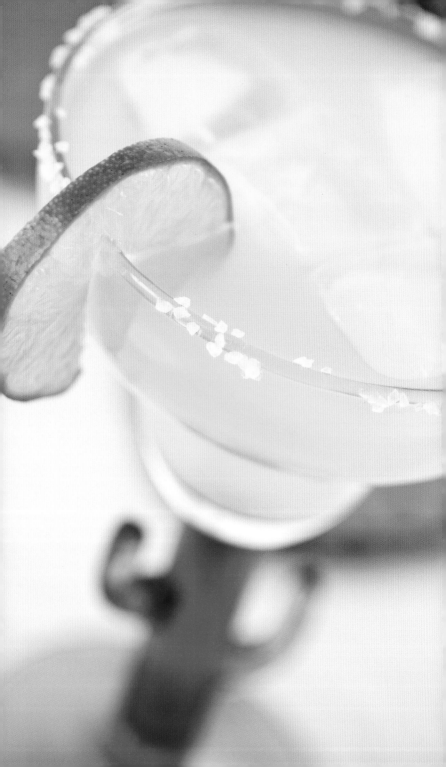

Stemware

Everything tastes better when sipped from the appropriate vessel! If you don't already have elegant stemware, this could be a great time to indulge. Holding a Preggatini in a beautiful glass makes you feel sexy, whether you're pregnant or not. I love scouring secondhand shops for vintage treasures. Gorgeous little cocktail glasses do not have to cost a fortune. If your grandma invites you to raid her china cabinet, even better. Obviously, drinks are not limited to the suggested stemware listed below. This guide corresponds to drinks throughout the following recipes and gives you an idea of what to buy for your home bar.

 BAR MUGS: These are thick, heat-resistant glass mugs used for cold or hot drinks.

COUPES: These are the original wide-mouthed champagne glasses that, according to legend, were molded from Queen Marie Antoinette's breast! Coupes allow for more aroma to escape than narrow flute glasses and encourage the little bubbles to tickle your nose. Many vintage cocktail glasses are a variation on a coupe.

MARTINI/COCKTAIL: V-shaped glasses

ROCKS/DOUBLE ROCKS: Short and stout glasses

COLLINS: These are tall, cylindrical glasses used for long drinks. A shorter version is called a highball glass.

WINE GLASSES: Stemware with a smaller, narrower bowl, used for white wine

WINE GOBLETS: Stemware that features a wider, rounder bowl and is used for red wine

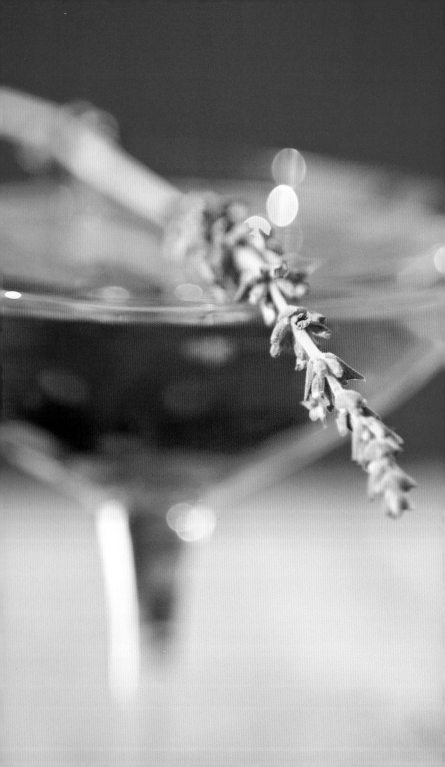

Kitchen Appliances

While the term *mixologist* is used to connote skilled bartenders who are trained in spirits and classic drinks, the term *bar chef* is also sometimes used and with good reason. Many bar programs require time in the kitchen to prepare syrups, purees, garnishes, and other culinary ingredients. These basic kitchen appliances will help you create Preggatinis on par with any professional cocktail bar.

BLENDER: For crushing ice and creating smoothie-style drinks

FOOD PROCESSOR: For grinding dry goods or quickly chopping fruits and vegetables

JUICER: Freshly juiced fruits and vegetables, rather than frozen or bottled, make mocktails unbelievably delicious and nutritious!

SAUCEPANS: For cooking syrups and purees

Stock Your Preggatini Bar

Skip the sugar rush (and subsequent headache) of sickly sweet "tini" drinks in favor of those with fresh, natural ingredients. Whether cooking, cocktail-making, or Preggatini mixing, balancing sweet, citrus, creamy, herbaceous, and spicy flavors just takes a little know-how, which you will learn in this book. These are some ingredients to keep on hand so you can whip up your favorite Preggatini whenever a craving strikes.

ACCESSORIES: Umbrellas, swizzle sticks, cocktail picks, coasters, colored reusable or compostable straws, mini clothespins, and basically anything fun to hang on the side of a glass will make your mocktail that much more special!

BITTERS: Heralded for their medicinal qualities, bitters have been used to settle minor gastric ailments for centuries. They are typically made by brewing herbs, roots, and/or bark in alcohol, although there are some bitters made in alcohol-free solutions. Using bitters is like using extracts in a cookie recipe: Only a couple of drops are added, and there is a range of flavors. If the alcohol in traditional bitters concerns you, check with your doctor before using them, and consider them an optional ingredient throughout this book.

DAIRY: Milk, whipping cream, half-and-half, and yogurt will make your drinks rich and creamy. There are also nondairy alternatives such as almond, coconut, oat, macadamia, and soy milks; coconut cream; and so on that will do the trick.

DRIED FLOWERS AND FLORAL WATERS: Dried lavender, jasmine, hibiscus flowers, orange flower, and rose waters are found at specialty culinary stores or online and provide subtle layers of flavor.

FRESH FRUIT, JUICES, AND NECTARS: Always buy fresh as needed when possible and use frozen or canned when they are out of season. Stock up on lemons, limes, oranges, grapefruits, pineapples, watermelons, cantaloupes, honeydews, mangoes, peaches, raspberries, blueberries, blackberries, cherries, pomegranates, apricots, guava nectar, tamarind nectar, acai puree, coconut water, lychees, grapes, and so on.

FRESH HERBS (BUY AS NEEDED): Fresh basil, dill, rosemary, cilantro, and thyme lend fresh aromatics and elevate drink making just as they do in cooking.

FRESH VEGGIES: Tomatoes, cucumbers, celery, carrots, beets, bell peppers, spinach, and so on make amazing juices, and usually have less sugar than fruit juices.

GARNISHES: Edible flowers, edible gold leaf, flavored and colored rimming sugars, candied ginger, dried or chocolate-covered fruits add extra pizzazz.

MIXERS: Club soda, ginger ale, ginger beer (it's nonalcoholic), tonic water, and flavored waters are bar staples.

QUALITY ICE: Large, solid cubes melt slowly so they don't water down the drink too quickly. Invest in a few ice cube trays with deep cavities, and use purified or filtered water for the best-tasting drinks. Also, try freezing juice, teas, mixers, decaf coffee, and other tasty liquids into ice cubes—as they melt, the drink becomes more flavorful.

SPICES: Fresh ginger, jalapeños, black pepper, cayenne pepper, Worcestershire sauce, horseradish, Tabasco, cloves, cinnamon sticks, nutmeg, and so on are featured in many recipes.

> "To get a great drink, start with quality ingredients. You can't build a Ferrari out of Ford parts."
> —TONY ABOU-GANIM, *THE MODERN MIXOLOGIST*

SIMPLE SYRUP *(to easily sweeten drinks)*

> 1 cup sugar (experiment with different kinds such as raw or brown to get different flavors from the syrup)

> 1 cup water

Heat sugar and water in a small saucepan. Stir until sugar dissolves. Cool and refrigerate.

More "sweet" suggestions:

- Add a tablespoon of grated ginger root, lavender, hibiscus, or a few hot chili peppers to the saucepan for flavored syrups.

- Layer flavor by substituting floral waters or flavored teas in place of plain water.

- Agave nectar can be substituted for simple syrup. And, to make a honey syrup, mix two parts honey with one part water.

SHRUBS

Shrubs are vinegar-based drinks that hearken back to colonial times. Preserving fruit in vinegar was a common way to store produce for the winter season. Once it sat for a while, pouring off a little of the vinegar solution into a glass, sweetening it, and diluting it with water made it a healthful drink. In recent years, shrubs have made a comeback as an ingredient in modern cocktails and mocktails. My basic shrub recipe includes about one part each of vinegar, sugar, and very ripe fruit. Because the sugar is already mixed in, you may not need to sweeten it further. Get creative by experimenting with different vinegars and fruits. Here are a few ideas to get you started.

CANTALOUPE AND STRAWBERRY SHRUB

> ¾ cup cantaloupe (peeled and seeded)
>
> ¾ cup strawberries (hulled)
>
> 1 cup apple cider vinegar
>
> 1 cup raw sugar

Place all ingredients in a blender for 10 to 15 seconds. Let mixture sit in the fridge overnight, then strain. Keep liquid in fridge for up to a week.

APRICOT AND LAVENDER SHRUB

> 1 cup apricots (halved, pits removed)
>
> 1 tablespoon dried culinary lavender
>
> 1 cup white vinegar
>
> 1 cup white granulated sugar

Place all ingredients in a blender for 10 to 15 seconds, just to mix them up. Let mixture sit in the fridge overnight, then strain. Keep liquid in fridge for up to a week.

MIXED BERRIES AND JALAPEÑO SHRUB

> 1 cup mixed berries (blackberries, raspberries, blueberries, and even cherries are great)
>
> 1 jalapeño (sliced and seeded)
>
> 1 cup balsamic vinegar
>
> 1 cup raw sugar

Place all ingredients in a blender for 10 to 15 seconds. Let mixture sit in the fridge overnight, then strain. Keep liquid in fridge for up to a week.

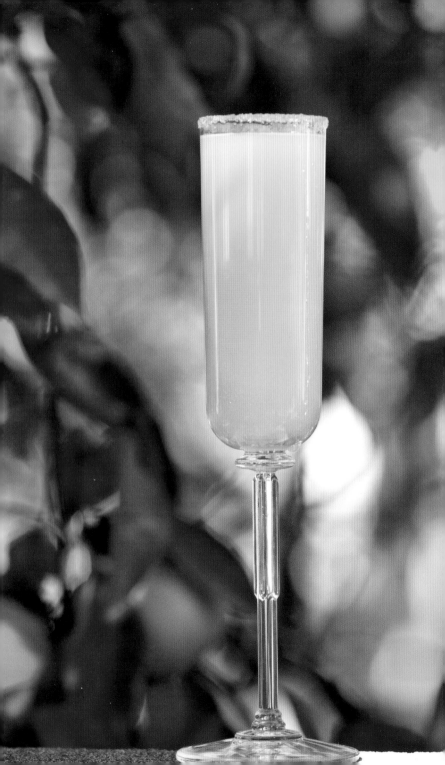

Part Two
An "Extra Kick" for Non-Preggie Pals

Nonalcoholic cocktails have become a worldwide trend, and people enjoy a quality booze-free drink whether they are pregnant or not. Preggatinis are designed to celebrate the mom-to-be, but I hope this book will remain a useful mixology guide long after your baby is delivered and the doctor says it is safe to drink alcohol again. Therefore, I have included simple directions throughout this book to turn these mocktails into cocktails with a flip of the jigger.

Despite some physical discomforts, such as a few well-placed kicks from a growing fetus, an expectant mom experiences the miraculous pregnancy journey in a way no one else can. Still, she is not the only one expecting a baby. They say it takes a village to raise a baby, and the village wants to share in the joy!

Some partners support through solidarity and lay off the sauce while Mama is growing a human. Others might want to keep on toasting with something from the liquor cabinet. It doesn't hurt to entice the Preggatini-tender to whip up a virgin drink for non-booze-drinkers, and then add a little "kick" to that same recipe for those who aren't abstaining.

There are some amazing alcohol-free alternatives that taste like gin or rum or whiskey as you'll see in recipes throughout this book. But first, this simple overview of basic spirits will guide non-preggie pals who want to add a kick to the recipes in this book. It also keeps these recipes relevant for all occasions in the years to come.

VODKA can be made from, well, anything. There are vodkas made from potatoes, fruits, grains, and even milk! It is (somewhat unfairly) defined as a "characterless" spirit, meaning it is the most versatile addition to any juicy mixture for your non-preggie pals looking for a boozy kick. Consider it the "chicken breast" of alcohol . . . it has a relatively bland flavor itself, so it goes with pretty much everything.

GIN is essentially flavored vodka. All gins must be infused with juniper, but apart from that, the other ingredients vary wildly. Classic London Dry style will be heavy on the juniper flavor and likely have some coriander, clove, or peppercorn added. A more modern approach to gin is lighter on the juniper and brings in fruity, floral notes.

TEQUILA is the most popular of the agave spirits. In order to be called "tequila," the spirit must be made from 100 percent Blue Webber Agave plant and can only be produced in Mexico. *Blanco* tequila is unaged, *reposado* means it has rested in a wood barrel for up to six months, and *añejo* indicates the liquid has aged in a barrel for up to a year. The liquid darkens the longer it is in the barrel. Avoid buying anything called "gold," as that usually means artificial color has been added rather than naturally derived through the wooden barrel. Another fun fact is that tequila is actually one kind of mezcal, which is a broad category of spirits made from various agave plants.

RUM is another broad category of spirits made predominantly from molasses or sugar. Rum comes in light, dark, spiced, and there's even a funky Rhum Agricole made in the Caribbean. Cachaca is a sugarcane spirit made in Brazil that is similar to rum but falls into its own category. Rums can be clear or aged in wood, just like some tequilas, whiskies, and brandies. It naturally has a slightly sweeter taste and is incredibly versatile. Non-preggie pals will want to try it in a variety of fruity, tropical drinks.

WHISK(E)Y is a huge spirits category because it is made all around the world. The most popular styles include Scotch, Bourbon, Rye, Irish, Canadian, and Japanese. Whiskey can be made from all kinds of grains and must be aged in barrels, which is how it gets its lovely amber color. Bourbon is the "sweetest" of the whiskies, as it is made from at least 51 percent corn. If you have a non-preggie pal looking to give their Preggatini a whiskey kick, they likely already know which style they prefer.

BRANDIES are made from fruit. The most famous ones—Cognac, Armagnac from France, Spanish brandy, and Chilean or Peruvian Pisco—are made from grapes. But brandies can also be made from cherries, apricots, and so on. These are also very versatile spirits and mix easily into many of the Preggatinis for non-pregnant friends, adding a little kick to their mocktail.

"Cocktails are sexy and play a leading role in the perfect courtship. Now the wedding is a distant but sweet memory and a new chapter is beginning in your lives: She is pregnant. It is a great feeling, the beginning of your family; so much lies ahead. Then Saturday night rolls around and you decide to stay at home and cook, cozy up in the nest. He makes himself a dry martini, and then it hits . . . what does she drink? Approach nonalcoholic cocktails with the same attention given their stronger cousins. Use good glassware and fresh ingredients, and garnish with style."

—Dale DeGroff, King Cocktail, the "Godfather" of modern mixology and author of *The Craft of the Cocktail*, among others. Wife Jill DeGroff is a famous saloon artist depicting beloved bars and mixology personalities around the world.

There are many other spirits to enjoy once the ban on booze is lifted after baby's arrival. I hope your favorite Preggatini recipes in this book will prove great cocktail bases when you're ready to dip your toe back into the tippling pond. Consider exploring Korean soju, Japanese sake, Chinese *baiju*, absinthe, liqueurs, and eau de vies of all sorts in your experimentation.

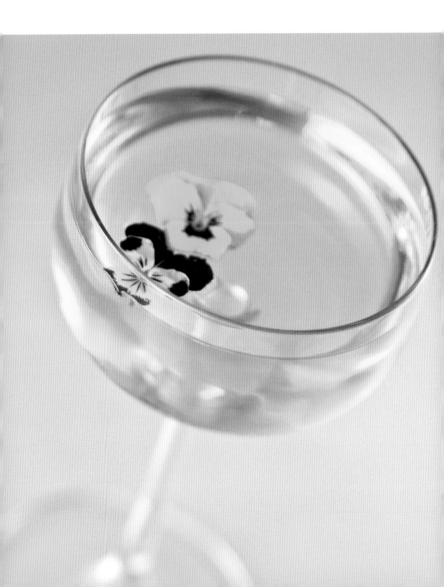

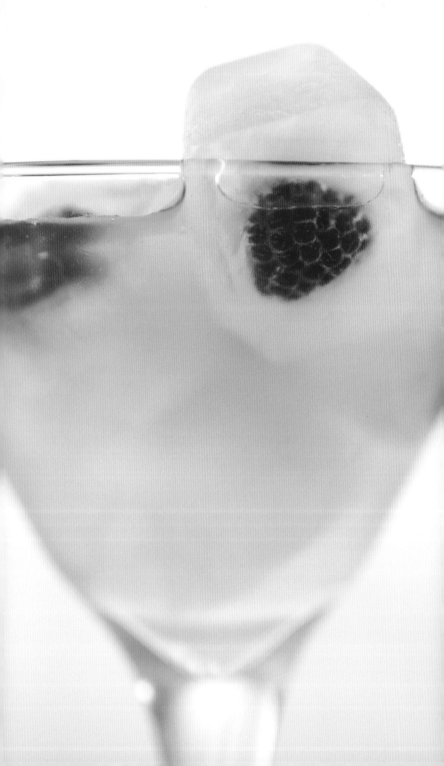

Part Three
Preggatinis: Let's Shake Things Up!

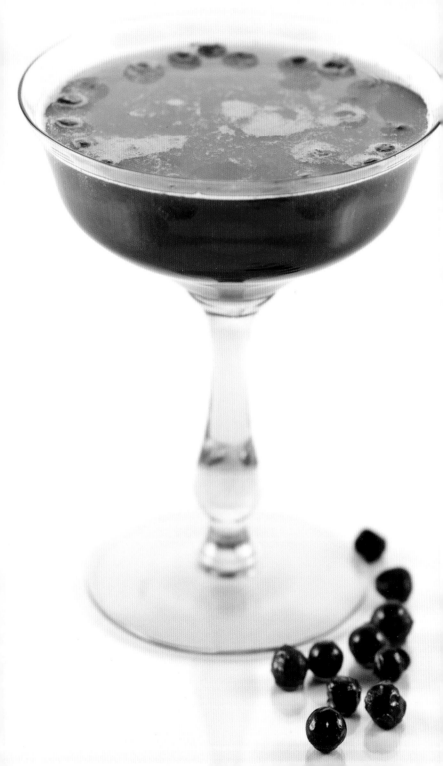

1

Pre-Pregnancy

Before you toss your wine glasses out the window in anticipation of a long, dry year ahead, rest assured that Preggatinis maintain all the fun, flavor, and fancy stemware of cocktail hour. Nowadays even the swankiest cocktail bars around the world include liquorless libations for people taking a break from booze. Thanks to the latest health trends, there has never been a better time to become a mocktail maven.

As you prepare your guest *womb* for its visitor, a little spring cleaning may be in order. Sure, have that last hurrah with a girls' night out and party like it's spring break before you start cooking a bun in the oven. But when you're serious about baby-making, start with the "detox" Preggatinis in this chapter to rinse out that liver, clear your mind, and load up on vitamins with fresh juices. Finally, when it's time to get down to the business of getting down, seal the deal with liquid aphrodisiacs. The last drink in this chapter is a soothing sipper called Anticipation, designed to quell your nerves while you await those home pregnancy test results.

Cleaning House

For the gals who want to "go big" before they "go bust," visit The Liquid Muse website for cocktail inspiration. But when you're ready to grow a baby, you need to prep your body from the inside out. Fresh fruits and veggies, lots of water, sunshine, fresh air, and prenatal vitamins help prepare a healthy environment for your little one. It's time to breathe, stretch, rest, and generally put prudence before partying. Treating your body like the temple it is will prepare it for a nice, long visit from you know who, and maintain your own self-care. There's a lot of excitement ahead, so let's start with a clean foundation.

 ## CLEAN AS A WHISTLE WITH MILK THISTLE
(Bar Mug)

Everything we eat—and drink—gets filtered through the liver. Milk thistle is the crucial ingredient of this warm tonic because it is thought to aid in liver detox. Fresh mint helps sooth digestion and promotes relaxation whether indulging in this elixir first thing in the morning or when snuggling up at night.

> 8 to 10 fresh mint leaves, plucked
>
> 1 milk thistle tea bag*
>
> 1 teaspoon wildflower honey (or to taste)
>
> 1 lemon wedge

Muddle the mint leaves in the bottom of a mug to extract the natural oils and flavor from the leaves. (Take a whiff, the smell of fresh mint is wonderfully soothing!) Add the milk thistle tea bag and pour in boiling water. Let it sit for about 5 minutes. Remove tea bag and mint, then stir in the honey until it dissolves. Garnish with lemon wedge.

If you may already be pregnant, double-check all herbal remedies with your doctor before ingesting.

INSIDE SPA
(Cocktail Glass)

Have you ever had cool, soothing cucumber slices placed on your eyes during a facial? Or sipped cucumber water while waiting for a massage at a spa? This refreshing cucumber concoction hydrates your baby-making organs from the inside out, and the cayenne pepper is believed to stimulate internal cleansing.

½ cucumber, peeled and seeded

¾ ounce lemon juice

1 tablespoon agave nectar

Pinch of ground cayenne pepper

Blend cucumber, lemon juice, and agave nectar until smooth. Pour mixture into a cocktail glass. Add sprinkle of cayenne pepper.

Extra Kick for Non-Preggie Pals: Add 1½ ounces cucumber-flavored vodka, or try tequila or gin.

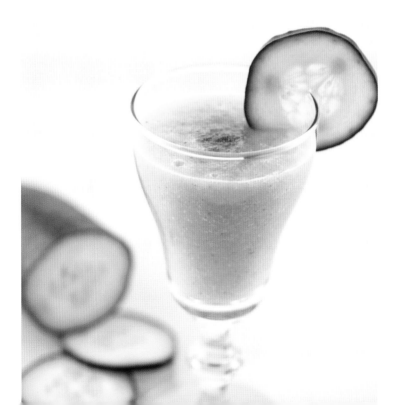

POMEGRANATE COOLER
(Collins Glass)

Pomegranates are packed with vitamin C, niacin, and iron. They have even been declared a "super fruit" by the media, including Oprah Winfrey, who is said to be fond of pomegranate martinis. Blueberries and grapes are also full of antioxidants, giving this cooler a one-two punch!

½ cup fresh or frozen blueberries

3 ounces pomegranate juice

2 ounces white grape juice

3 ounces berry-flavored sparkling water

1 lemon slice

Muddle the blueberries in the bottom of a Collins glass. Then add ice and pour in the juices. Fill the glass to the top with sparkling water and place a lemon slice on top of the drink. Sip through a colorful straw.

Extra Kick for Non-Preggie Pals: Along with the juices, add 1½ ounces of any clear spirit.

ACCORDING TO GREEK LORE, Persephone (the sunny-dispositioned daughter of Zeus) is forced to spend four months each year in the underworld because she could not resist the temptation of eating seeds from a forbidden pomegranate. During her absence the earth becomes cold and barren—in other words, this is the Ancient Greek explanation for winter.

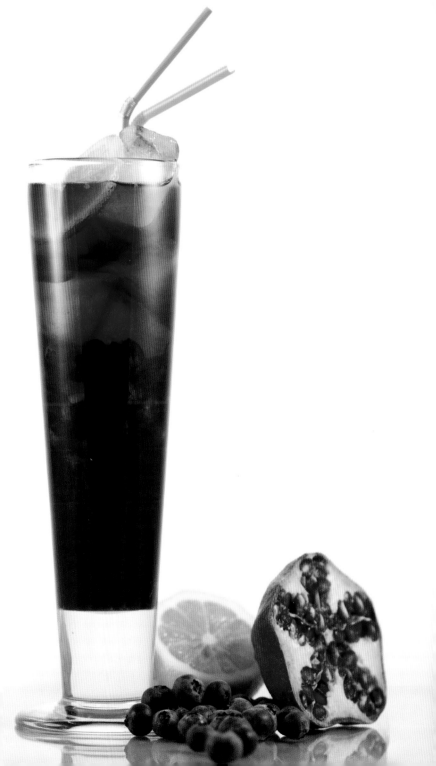

Getting Down to Business

Okay, so your body is not only a temple, it's also a pleasure palace! Some would argue that the best part of being pregnant is getting pregnant. This next round of non-boozy-floozie drinks is designed to keep you and your man up to the task of baby-making. Drawing from a range of touted aphrodisiacs, these Preggatinis help get the private party started. Brew some passion potions in your cauldron of seduction so when ovulation strikes, you can enjoy a delicious nonalcoholic drink and have a darn good time in the process.

 ## SWEET NOTHINGS
(Champagne Flute)

If your guy is the romantic type, this cocktail may set the stage for a soirée d'amour. Remember, you can spike his with real sparkling wine if you think he may need a little liquid encouragement.

> 3 ounces nonalcoholic sparkling wine
>
> 1½ ounces orange juice
>
> 1½ ounces mango juice (or nectar)
>
> 1 maraschino cherry

Pour the nonalcoholic sparkling wine into a champagne flute. Gently add the juices. Garnish with maraschino cherry, and test your partner's talents by seeing if they can tie the stem in a knot with their tongue.

OYSTER SHOT
(Rocks Glass)

If you've ever been on a hot date at a seafood restaurant, you may have shared a secret giggle when ordering oysters. Long rumored to be a mouthful of hot lovin' aphrodisiac, oysters are high in zinc, which is said to boost progesterone levels . . . electrifying the libido.

½ ounce lemon juice

2 ounces tomato juice

Dash of Worcestershire sauce

Smidge of horseradish

1 plump, juicy oyster, shucked*

Shake all liquid ingredients with ice. Pour into a glass. Plop in the oyster. Sip, slurp, and spice up your evening!

*If you may already be pregnant, check with your doctor before eating raw seafood.

Extra Kick for Non-Preggie Pals:
Add an ounce of vodka with the other liquids.

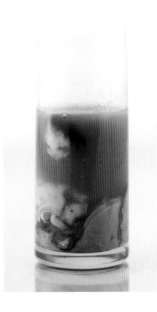

PANTS ON FIRE
(Martini Glass)

Ignite a night of hot passion by sipping a nonalcoholic cocktail with a kick! This spicy tipple includes lust-inducing chili and passion fruit, which is said to have a calming effect. Perfect for a relaxing-yet-exciting night in.

> **3 ounces passion fruit juice**
>
> **3 ounces guava nectar**
>
> **¾ ounce chili-infused Simple Syrup (recipe page 10)**
>
> **1 teaspoon grenadine**
>
> **1 small Thai chili**

Pour passion fruit puree, juices, and chili-infused syrup into a mixing glass. Shake with ice. Strain into a chilled martini glass. Gently pour prickly pear syrup into the drink, allowing it to settle at the bottom of the glass. Garnish with a Thai chili on a toothpick on the side of the glass.

Extra Kick for Non-Preggie Pals: Place a few hot chilis in a bottle of vodka. Let sit for a few days. The spirit will have absorbed flavor and spice from the pods—and it will keep getting hotter over time! Shake 1 ounce of the fiery vodka along with the juices and simple syrup.

> SPICY FOODS act as an aphrodisiac and are even said to rev up the metabolism. So get the party started—and keep it going—with chili!

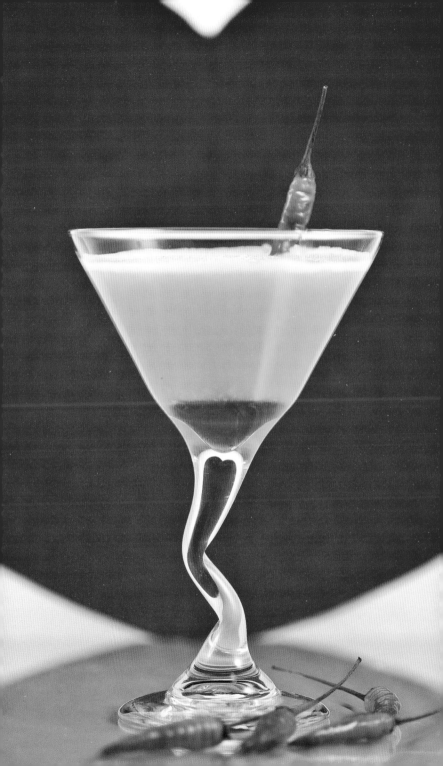

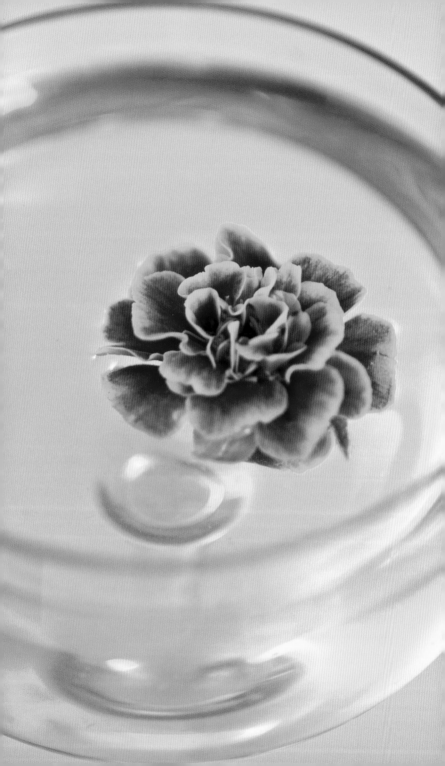

Drum Roll, Please

After all that hard work, it's time for the moment of truth. Did you conceive, or are you sentenced to another month of hot sex with your partner? (If you're not in a hurry to get pregnant, this could be a winning situation however you look at it.) No matter what the result, taking a pregnancy test can be a nerve-wracking experience, so here's a drink to sooth your nerves.

ANTICIPATION
(Cocktail Glass)

You bought the box. You did the awkward "wetting of the stick." Now you wait. It may be only a few minutes, but it can feel like forever. Here's something to keep your mind, and your taste buds, occupied.

> **5 to 6 ounces brewed chamomile tea**
>
> **2 teaspoons wildflower honey**
>
> **½ ounce lemon juice**
>
> **1 edible flower**

Pour warm brewed tea into a mixing glass. Stir in the wildflower honey then add the lemon juice. Add ice, shake, then strain into a chilled cocktail glass. Garnish with edible flower.

DID YOU KNOW that cocktail glasses originally held only 4 or 5 ounces of liquid? That's about half the size of what is used in today's bars, many of which serve 8- to 12-ounce martinis. (No wonder we wake up with pounding heads!)

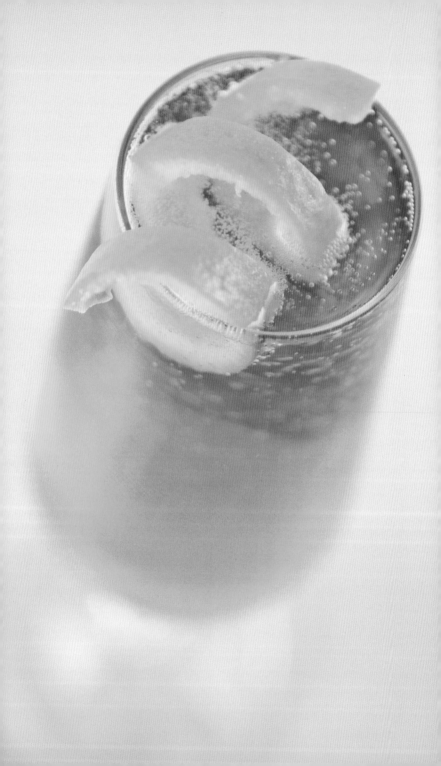

2

First Trimester

Congratulations, you got knocked up! Whether this is your first baby or your fifth, a long-cherished dream or a (gulp) wonderful surprise, both egg and sperm can rightfully declare "Mission Accomplished." It's time to celebrate your ability to procreate. You're about to welcome a baby into your life, the threshold of which is your uterus!

A Bun in the Oven

Your body is now your baby's temple. Even though you may be puking up your decaf lattes these first few months of pregnancy, it is important to incorporate extra nutrients into your diet. This chapter addresses worshipping yourself, and your thriving reproductive system, as the fertile goddess you are!

These drinks are perfect for a little impregnation celebration, to ease morning sickness, and I've included several fanciful drinks filled with folic acid, which is integral to fetal development during the first trimester. Nothing says "Whoopee!" like clinking glasses to punctuate the occasion and toasting a job well done.

 ## THREE'S COMPANY
(Collins Glass)

A baby transforms a couple into a family. It is a living, breathing expression of the love and deepens already profound bonds. In other words, this third wheel is a welcome addition.

> **3 thinly sliced lemon wheels**
>
> **3 ounces pink lemonade**
>
> **3 ounces lemon soda (bitter lemon soda is best if you can find it!)**
>
> **3 strawberries**

Fill a Collins glass with ice. Line the glass with lemon slices. Pour in pink lemonade and lemon soda. Garnish with three strawberries on a cocktail skewer laid across the top of the glass.

Extra Kick for Non-Preggie Pals: Add an ounce of citrus-flavored vodka or limoncello, a sweet Italian lemon liqueur.

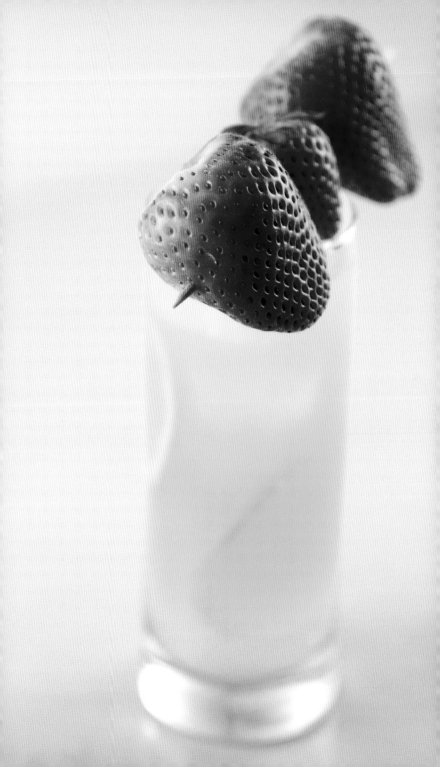

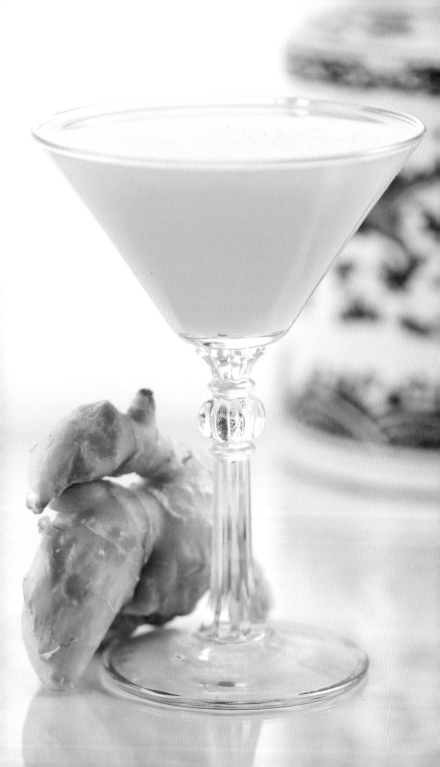

THE MORNING AFTER
(Martini Glass)

Normally, if you woke up feeling queasy after a big celebration, you might drink a lot of water, take an aspirin, and have a nice, long nap until the alcohol worked itself out of your system. However, as much as I hate to bring it up, you may be worshipping the porcelain god for a couple of months—and it has nothing to do with liquor. Luckily, ginger is nature's answer to an upset tummy and morning sickness, clove is an ancient remedy for staving off nausea, and the vinegar in the apricot and lavender shrub can help restore the pH balance in the stomach.

- 1 cup sugar (experiment with different kinds of sugar)
- 1 cup water
- 1 tablespoon grated ginger root
- 1 ounce Apricot and Lavender Shrub (recipe page 11)
- 3 ounces apricot nectar
- Pinch of ground clove

Make your simple syrup first by heating the sugar, water, and ginger root in a small saucepan. Stir until sugar dissolves. Cool and refrigerate.

Shake remaining ingredients plus ¾ ounce of the ginger-infused simple syrup with ice, then strain into a martini glass.

Extra Kick for Non-Preggie Pals: Add 1½ ounces of vodka or gin.

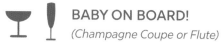

BABY ON BOARD!
(Champagne Coupe or Flute)

For the next nine months, wherever you go, so goes baby. Your tummy is a taxi whose passenger has settled in for the ride of a lifetime. Instinct makes you extra cautious with every move, so isn't it fun to know that drinking Preggatinis while hauling this cargo isn't hazardous in the least?

3 ounces mango nectar

1 ounce lime juice

2 ounces lime-flavored sparkling water

1 maraschino cherry

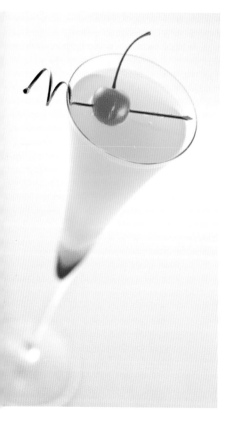

Pour mango nectar, lime juice, and sparkling water into a champagne coupe or flute. Garnish with a maraschino cherry on a pick across the edge of the glass.

PREGGIE PARADISE
(Rocks Glass)

Preparing to meet your baby is one of the happiest times of your life, despite any temporary queasiness! Lift a glass to your little angel. (Bonus: Bitters help settle a queasy stomach!)

- **1 ounce pineapple juice**
- **Orange bitters**
- **3 ounces ginger beer**
- **1 pineapple wedge**

Pour ingredients into a rocks glass filled with ice. Garnish with a pineapple wedge on the edge of the glass.

Extra Kick for Non-Preggie Pals: Add 1½ ounces rum.

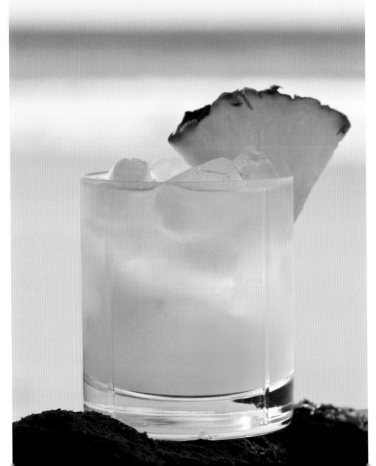

Frolicking with Folic Acid

Folic acid, also known as folate, is one of the building blocks of life and an integral nutrient during the first few months of pregnancy. By now you're taking prenatal vitamins, which are meant to supplement folate, calcium, and iron during this crucial time in your baby's early development. The following drinks support that effort with ingredients such as cantaloupe, kiwi, berries, papaya, spinach, and beets.

FOLIC FIZZ
(Wine Glass)

Cantaloupe's folic quotient makes it among the best choices for First Trimester Preggatinis. This one is punctuated with iron-rich strawberries to make it extra tasty and good for you.

> 2 to 3 ounces Cantaloupe and Strawberry Shrub (recipe page 11)
>
> Club soda
>
> 1 strawberry (sliced)

Pour shrub and club soda into a wine glass and add a few ice cubes if desired. Add strawberries.

Extra Kick for Non-Preggie Pals: Add 1½ ounces of vodka, gin, or tequila.

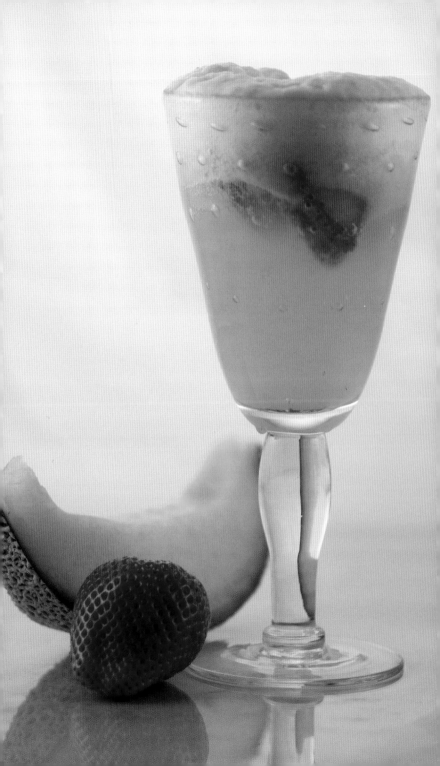

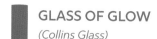

GLASS OF GLOW
(Collins Glass)

Are people already starting to mention how radiant you look? In addition to hormonal surges, your glow comes from taking better care of yourself. Just consider pregnancy nature's way of making you even more beautiful.

3 to 5 ripe blackberries

1 kiwi (peeled)

6 ounces coconut water

Slice of kiwi

Gently muddle the blackberries and kiwi in the bottom of a mixing glass. Add coconut water and ice. Shake well then strain into a tall, ice-filled glass. Slide a slice of kiwi onto the rim of the glass.

FRUITY FOLATE SHAKE
(Collins Glass)

Papayas are loaded with folate, and bananas are high in potassium. Add a swirl of sweet coconut milk, and this blended Preggatini is a great boost of energy any time of the day.

½ cup fresh papaya chunks (or ⅓ cup papaya nectar)

½ banana

½ cup coconut milk

4 ice cubes

Pinch of grated coconut

Blend ingredients until smooth. Pour into a tall Collins glass. Sprinkle with grated coconut.

Extra Kick for Non-Preggie Pals: Add 1½ ounces coconut-flavored vodka or rum into the blender.

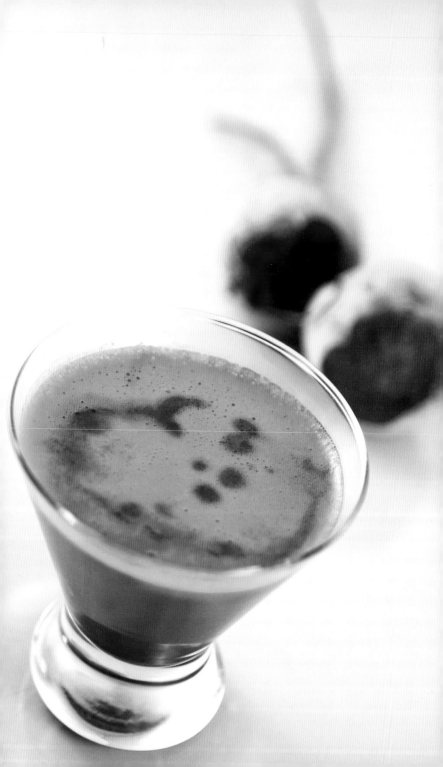

FEEL THE (HEART) BEET
(Double Rocks Glass)

By the end of the first trimester, you will hear your baby's heartbeat. This drink includes spinach—high in iron to fortify the red blood cells pulsing through your umbilical cord—as well as beets and carrots, which are full of vitamin C and folic acid. They're also high in sugar, so no extra sweetener is needed.

> **3 carrots, washed and peeled**
>
> **½ cup spinach**
>
> **1 beet, washed and peeled**

To create a layered effect in the glass, juice each vegetable separately, and gently pour the liquids into a rocks glass one at a time. The colorful combination is pleasing to the eye as well as the palate! If you are looking to consume extra fiber, liquify the veggies in an electric blender on high until smooth instead of juicing.

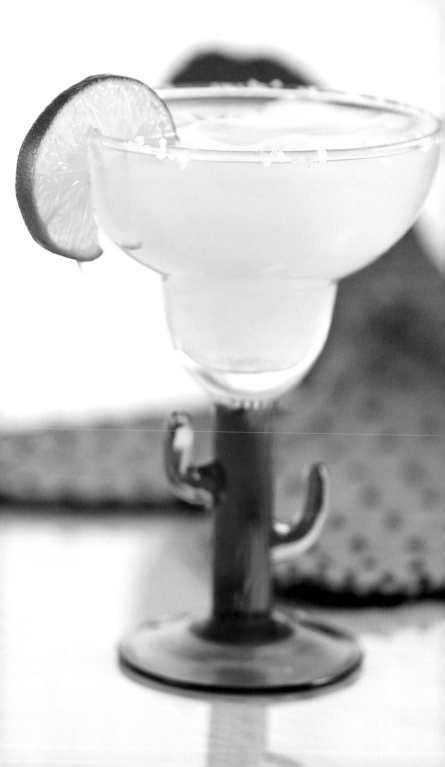

3

Second Trimester

Many newly pregnant moms decide to wait until the second trimester to sing their good news from the rooftops. And when they do, everyone wants to wish them well. Over the next few months, you will hear "Congratulations" so many times that you might (almost) get sick of it!

Although this book is filled with festive drink recipes to make at home . . . what do you do when you go out? Never fear. The first section of this chapter highlights cocktail menu alternatives and tells you how to order them so any well-heeled bartender will know exactly what you want. Plus, there are so many nonalcoholic spirits alternatives now that it's easy to re-create some of your favorite classic cocktails at home.

The biggest celebration of this trimester may be a special escape for parents-to-be . . . the babymoon! It's a chance to get away from the hullabaloo and stay up all night doing what got you pregnant in the first place, before you're up all night changing diapers. The Preggatinis in the third section of this chapter set the mood for that final fling, whether you're at a seaside resort or in a snowy chalet—or just snuggled up at home with the blinds down.

Belly Up to the Bar

As you transition from barfly to baby mama, you may wonder what to order during the next girls' night out. You won't feel like a wallflower while all your girlfriends are clinking colorful, tasty drinks in pretty glasses with these nonalcoholic cocktails you can order from any bartender and sound like a pro! Besides, booze-free options are finally catching on in restaurants. There are many "virgin spirits" on liquor store shelves, too, so you can be the MIXtress of your own liquid pleasure and turn your favorite classic cocktails into Preggatinis.

MADRAS MIA
(Collins Glass)

A Madras is vodka with cranberry and orange juices. It is a basic highball that any bartender can easily make without vodka, as cranberry and orange juice are behind every bar.

> 2½ ounces cranberry juice
>
> 2½ ounces orange juice
>
> Splash of club soda
>
> 1 lemon wedge

Pour all liquid ingredients into a tall Collins glass filled with ice. Garnish with a lemon wedge on the rim of the glass.

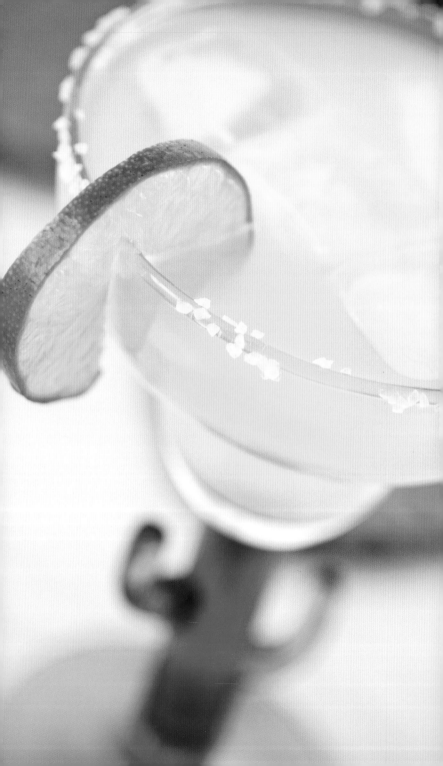

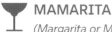

MAMARITA
(Margarita or Martini Glass)

Can't imagine a platter of sizzling fajitas without a margarita? This Preggatini version of your favorite Mexican concoction will have you dancing to the beat of your own mariachis! And instead of plain salt, this glass rimmer is equally sweet with an optional spicy suggestion.

1 lime

Kosher salt mixed with equal parts sugar (for an extra kick, add ground red chili powder)

2 ounces nonalcoholic tequila

¾ ounce orange juice

½ ounce fresh lime juice

½ ounce agave nectar

Lime wheel

Moisten half the rim of a glass with a cut lime, then dip it into spiced salt mixture and set aside. Shake remaining ingredients with ice and gently strain into the half-rimmed glass. Slide lime wheel onto rim of glass.

PHOTOGRAPH YOUR BEAUTIFUL BELLY. Schedule your own belly-centric photo shoot—maybe paint your belly, decorate it with flower garlands, or wear a special outfit that shows it off—and frame your favorite shot for the baby's room.

COSMOM
(Martini Glass)

The Cosmopolitan is considered a modern classic cocktail after gaining popularity in the 1990s. Associated with Madonna in her early years, and the fashionable *Sex in the City* television series, this "Like a Virgin" version of the Cosmo is a sip of kitsch cool with a chaser of delicious nostalgia.

2 ounces nonalcoholic vodka

¾ ounce orange juice

½ ounce lime juice

¾ ounce cranberry juice

1 lime twist

Shake ingredients with ice. Strain into a martini glass. Lay the lime twist on the rim of the glass.

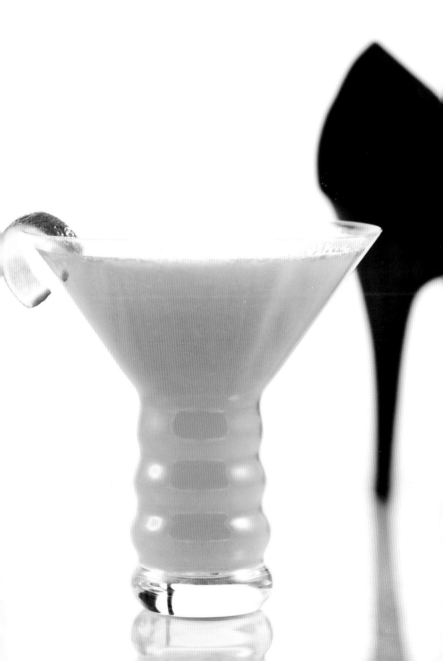

MAKE MINE A MOMJITO!
(Double Rocks Glass)

If the Latin cocktail craze has hit your 'hood, then you've probably sampled myriad creative incarnations of the mojito. This one stays close to a traditional recipe—only without the rum.

> 1 lime, quartered with peel on
>
> 6 to 8 mint leaves
>
> 1 teaspoon raw sugar
>
> 2 ounces nonalcoholic spiced rum
>
> Splash lemon-lime soda
>
> Sprig of mint

Muddle lime, mint, and sugar in the bottom of a glass. Add nonalcoholic spiced rum and lemon-lime soda. Fill with ice. Garnish with sprig of mint.

KING OF HEARTS NEGRONI
(Double Rocks Glass)

Negronis are one of my favorite classic cocktails, but it is all alcohol! Thank goodness there are some amazing nonalcoholic versions of spirits we love on store shelves—and in many bars—all around the world. I love adding grapefruit juice to regular Negronis, so I'm including it in this version.

1 ounce nonalcoholic gin

1 ounce nonalcoholic sweet vermouth

1 ounce nonalcoholic bitter liqueur (Campari substitute)

1 ounce grapefruit juice

Lemon twist or lime wheel

Shake ingredients with ice. Strain over fresh ice in a double rocks glass. Slip a lemon twist or lime wheel onto the rim of the glass.

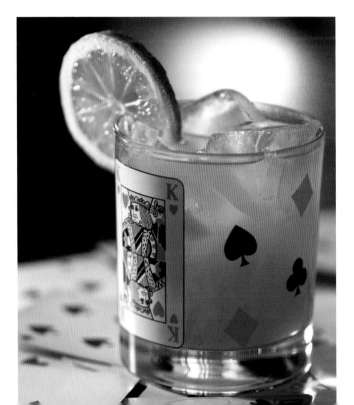

Babymoon Libations

Sometimes, parents-to-be snag a little "us" time with one last romantic getaway before baby arrives. Even if circumstances don't allow you to fly the coop before the stork delivers your little chick-a-dee, you can indulge in a date night themed around your fantasy trip. Dreaming of a tropical beach? Or maybe you envision warming each other up in a winter wonderland. Book an escape at your home bar!

 ### SAND BETWEEN OUR TOES
(Collins Glass)

You'll practically feel island breezes with every sip of this tropical treat. This recipe is enough for two, so warm up those coconuts and prepare to get lei-d!

- 3 ounces nonalcoholic rum
- 6 ounces pineapple juice
- 3 ounces coconut cream
- 2 ounce orgeat syrup (almond flavor)
- Slices of pineapple
- Colorful edible flowers

Blend all ingredients with ice. Pour into glasses and add beautiful garnishes.

HOT BUTTERED MUM'S RUM
(Bar Mug)

This Preggatini takes off the chill on a snowy evening and is the perfect complement to buttering up your loved one in front of a roaring fire.

1 cup water

Pinch of ground clove

½ ounce lemon juice

2 ounces Torani Butter Rum syrup

1 cinnamon stick

1 pat butter

Heat water, cloves, and lemon juice in a small saucepan, then pour into a bar mug. Add butter rum syrup, and garnish with a cinnamon stick and pat of butter.

Extra Kick for Non-Preggie Pals: Add an ounce of rum.

WHITE HOT MAMA
(Bar Mug)

Snuggle up and revel in your preggie fabulousness with this creamy glass of decadence with a kick. You're about to join the society of hot moms!

2 tablespoons caramel sauce

1 cup whole milk or nondairy milk

½ ounce chili-infused Simple Syrup (recipe page 10)

3 heaping tablespoons white hot chocolate powder

Drizzle caramel sauce around the inside of a bar mug. Heat milk in a small saucepan and mix in white hot chocolate powder and chili-infused syrup. Allow to cool slightly and then gently pour into the mug.

Extra Kick for Non-Preggie Pals: Add 1 ounce brandy, rum, whiskey, or aged tequila to the mixture.

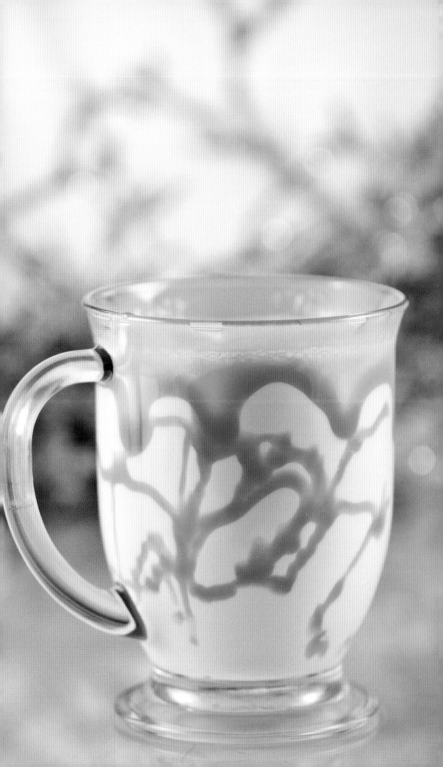

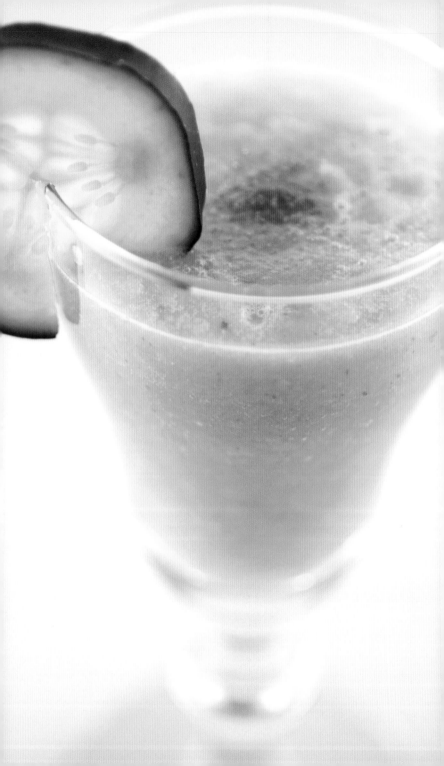

4

Third Trimester

Living large has never been more in fashion. The bigger your baby bump becomes, the more pregnant lady "street cred" you carry. There ain't no hiding it—so use it to your advantage! This chapter honors your special status, celebrates the little person you're about to meet, and offers some sweet relief for the last few weeks of pregnancy, which—let's face it—can be a little uncomfortable. Amid all the excitement, planning, and preparations for baby, don't forget to stop and smell the roses. You're about to be someone's mommy.

Pregnant and Proud!

Being a woman never feels more special than when you're flaunting your status as an integral link in perpetuating humanity. People offer you their seats on public transportation, hold open doors, and are only too happy to carry things for you. It's like stepping into an alternate universe filled with chivalrous knights at every turn. (Enjoy it while you can!) These drinks pay tribute to this moment in time, when every woman is entitled to a little extra-special attention.

 ## CALL ME PRINCESS PREGGATINI
(Martini Glass)

Have you ever played Queen for a Day? Well, being preggers, you get to play it every day for the better part of a year. Here's to you, Your Highness!

> ½ cup milk or nondairy milk
>
> 2 tablespoons strawberry milk powder or syrup
>
> 1 ounce grenadine
>
> Whipped cream or nondairy topping
>
> Red sprinkles

Pour milk and strawberry flavoring into a mixing glass and shake with ice. Gently add mixture to martini glass. Slowly drizzle in the grenadine, allowing it to sink to the bottom. Spoon on the whipped cream so that it becomes the top layer. Add red sprinkles, and serve alongside a rhinestone-encrusted tiara, of course!

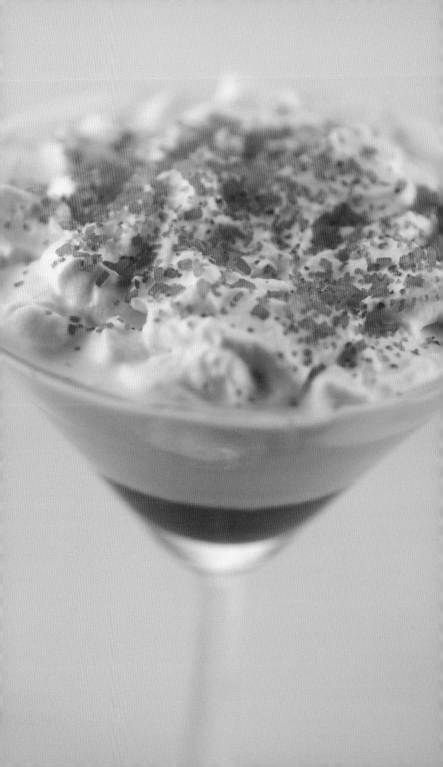

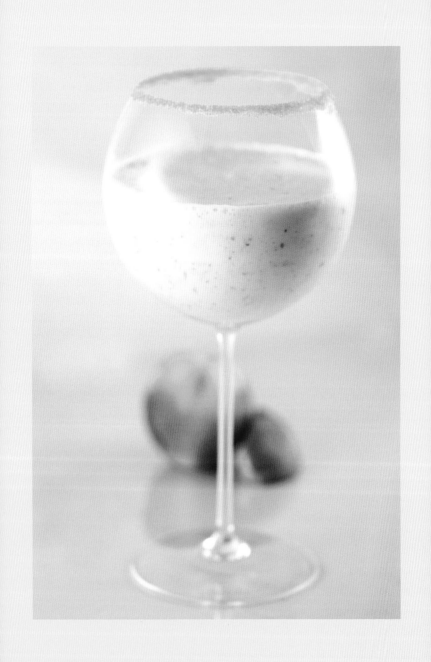

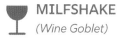

MILFSHAKE
(Wine Goblet)

A woman is most attractive when she is living in her power, and being a mom is one of the most powerful roles you will play in your life. Strong and nurturing, resilient and kind, moms are beautiful inside and out. And just because you're a grown woman with a kiddo (or three) doesn't mean you're any less of a fantasy girl.

> Flavored rimming sugar
>
> ½ cup peaches
>
> ¾ cup apricot nectar
>
> 1 scoop vanilla ice cream

Moisten the rim of a wine goblet, dip it into flavored sugar, and set aside. Blend the other ingredients and pour into the wine goblet.

Hello in There!

Although you may have a preference toward a daughter or a son, once your sonogram reveals who is kicking around inside your belly, you won't be able to imagine him or her any other way. For those of you who skip the surprise factor to start decorating, shopping for clothes, and picking names, here are some options for you.

 ## SWEET-N-SASSY
(Martini Glass)

Someday your adorable little angel will hit her teen years and become your biggest challenge. Driving lessons, first heartbreak, BFFs, and frenemies . . . so much drama! There will be plenty of reasons to pace the floor at night later in her life. Be thankful for these first few months when you pace the floor with her safely in your arms.

> Powdered sugar
>
> 3 ounces nonalcoholic rosé wine
>
> ½ ounce lemon juice
>
> 1 ounce raspberry syrup
>
> Three raspberries

Rim a martini glass with powdered sugar and set aside. Shake remaining ingredients with ice. Gently strain into the martini glass and serve with raspberries on a skewer.

Extra Kick for Non-Preggie Pals: Use a dry rosé wine and Chambord liqueur instead of raspberry syrup.

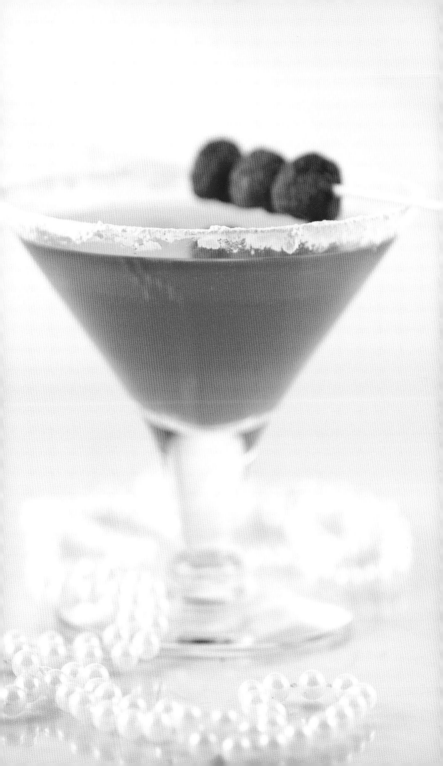

DOUBLE TROUBLE
(Double Rocks Glass)

Sometimes when people decide to start a family, they get lucky and conceive right away. And sometimes they get more than they bargained for . . . The first ingredient in this easy Preggatini is loaded with seven antioxidant-rich fruits to help you store up all the vitality you can.

3 ounces acai juice

2 ounces black cherry soda

Lemon wheel

Pour juice into an ice-filled double rocks glass, then top with black cherry soda. Stir to mix, and slide lemon wheel onto glass.

LITTLE BOY BLUE
(Champagne Coupe)

It's time to reacquaint yourself with nursery rhymes that make tiny tots coo. "Little Boy Blue" is a staple among baby's first forays into literature, and this drink may become a regular among your forays into Preggatinis.

3 ounces blueberry pomegranate juice

½ ounce lemon juice

¾ ounce blue pea flower tea Simple Syrup (recipe page 10)

Splash of club soda

3 blueberries

Shake juices and syrup with ice. Strain into a champagne coupe and top with club soda. Garnish with blueberries, loose or on a cocktail pick.

Extra Kick for Non-Preggie Pals: Add 1½ ounces berry-flavored vodka.

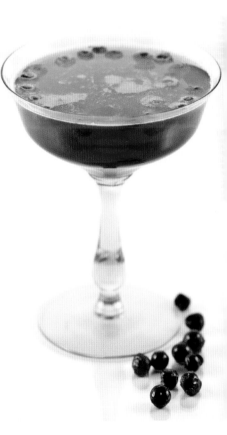

Easy Does It

As the arrival of your little one approaches, give yourself permission to take it easy. By the end of this trimester, you may have trouble sleeping, have bizarre cravings, or just feel slightly off-balance. These Preggatinis are intended to help ease physical discomforts as the big moment draws near.

SLEEPING BEAUTY
(Bar Mug)

A soothing glass of warm milk can help you relax before bed. Adding a swirl of honey and a sprinkle of cinnamon helps you catch a few winks of beauty sleep with a tasty treat in your tummy.

>   Cinnamon sugar (equal parts cinnamon and sugar)
>
>   1 cup whole or nondairy milk
>
>   2 teaspoons honey
>
>   1 teaspoon plus 1 pinch ground cinnamon, divided

Rim a bar mug with cinnamon sugar and set aside. Heat remaining ingredients in a small saucepan and let simmer for a few minutes on low heat. Pour into a bar mug. Sprinkle with a pinch of ground cinnamon.

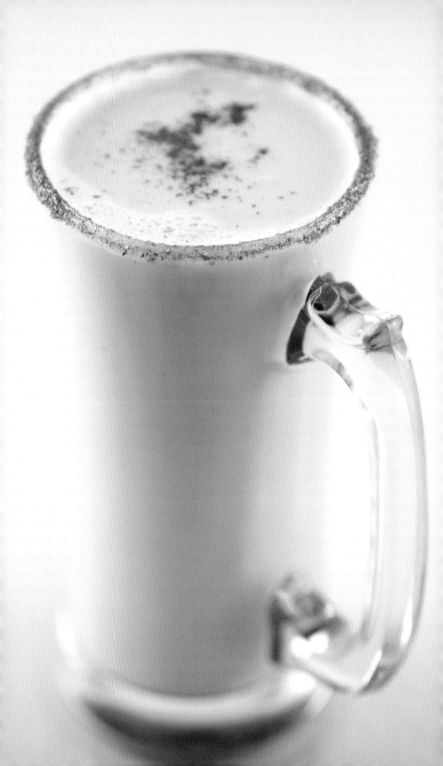

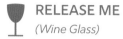

RELEASE ME
(Wine Glass)

As baby takes up more space, it is common to find some bodily functions temporarily interrupted. The mixture of delicious figs and prunes will help get things moving again!

3 fresh purple figs

1 ounce lavender Simple Syrup (recipe page 10)

4 ounces prune juice

Blend all ingredients until smooth. Strain into a wine glass—and don't travel too far from home for the next few hours!

FUNKY MONKEY
(Martini Glass)

The old cliché about fancying pickles and ice cream while pregnant may not be too far off base! Here is something to satisfy those odd cravings should they suddenly arise.

- **1 scoop chocolate ice cream**
- **½ banana**
- **1 tablespoon peanut butter**
- **½ cup whole or nondairy milk**
- **Whipped cream**
- **1 cherry**
- **2 pickles**

Blend ice cream, banana, peanut butter, and milk until smooth. Pour into a martini glass. Top with whipped cream and cherry. Serve with a side of pickles.

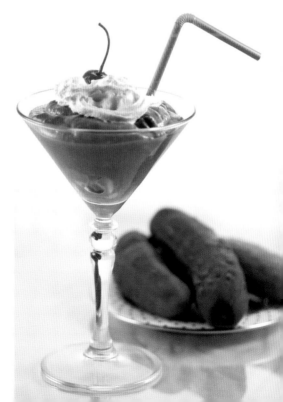

And Finally . . .

This Preggatini encourages you to take a moment for yourself in the days leading up to meeting the love of your life . . . your child.

 ## GARDEN ROSE
(Champagne Coupe)

Hopefully you've had a chance to sit quietly during this precious time and think about what motherhood means to you. As your belly unfurls into full bloom, budding within you is the beautiful, sacred, fragile gift of life.

> 1 heaping tablespoon diced cucumber (peeled and seeded)
>
> 1 ounce rose water Simple Syrup (recipe page 10)
>
> 3 ounces nonalcoholic Chardonnay
>
> Splash club soda
>
> 1 rose petal

Gently muddle cucumber and Rose Water Syrup in the bottom of a mixing glass. Add ice and wine, then shake well. Strain into a champagne coupe. Top with club soda. Garnish with a rose petal.

Extra Kick for Non-Preggie Pals: Substitute a favorite Chardonnay to make a wine cocktail, or use 1½ ounces vodka, gin, or tequila.

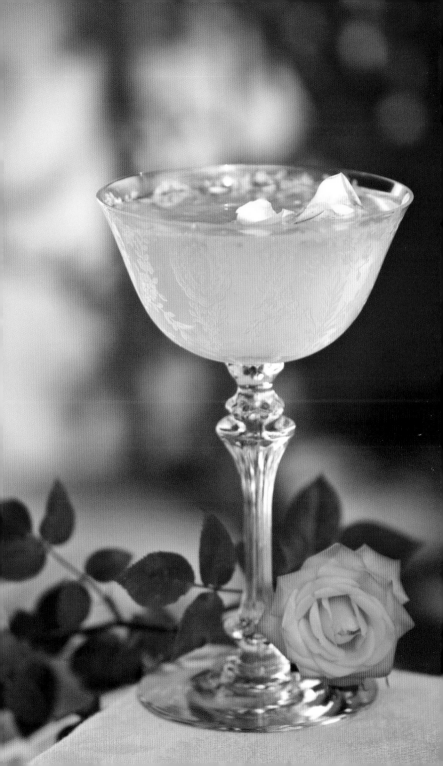

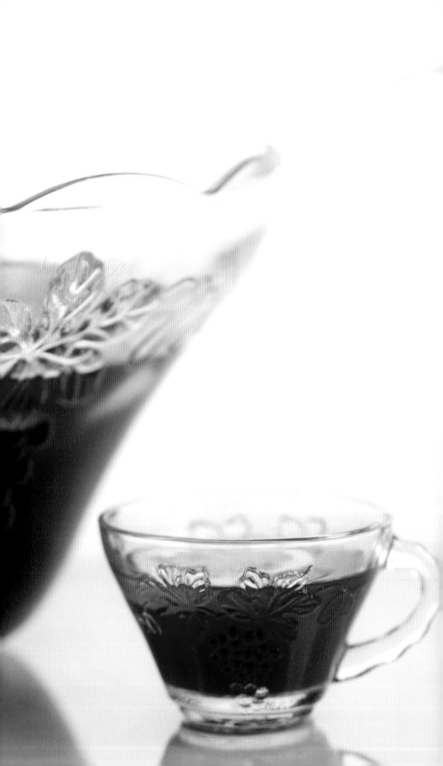

5

The Preggatini Party

Customized to fit the personality of the future mama, a Preggatini Party is a spiffed-up, modern celebration, designed to blow away a run-of-the-mill baby shower. Nonalcoholic cocktails for the guest of honor bring a hip vibe to the time-treasured gathering of family and friends, turning it into one of the most talked about social events of the year!

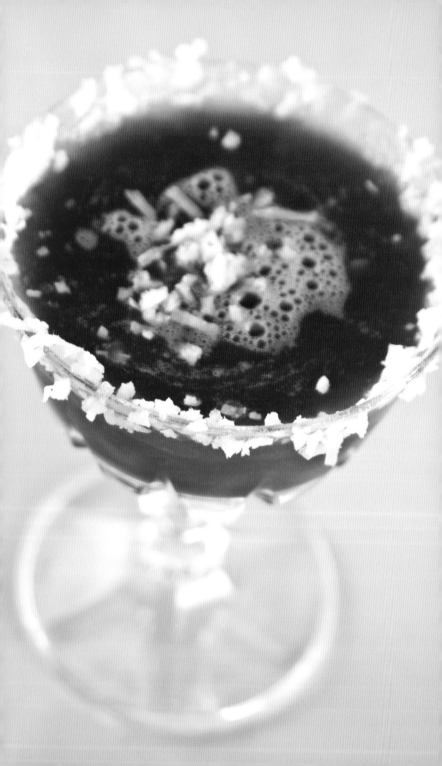

Party Like a Rock Star with CelebriBaby Preggatinis

Now that you've become a member of the child-bearing jet set, toast the star in your life (your baby) with a Preggatini to fit your own celebrity status. Invite your friends and fan club to raise a glass and step into the spotlight.

 ## POP PRINCESS
(Champagne Coupe)

You'll be ready to take center stage and party 'til you pop with this vitamin-packed mocktail. Tropical flavors and good-for-you ingredients will have you craving this drink long after your little one arrives.

- Ginger syrup
- Coconut flakes
- 3 ounces coconut water
- 3 ounces acai juice
- ¾ ounce ginger syrup
- ½ ounce lime juice

Dip the rim of the glass into a little ginger syrup poured onto a saucer, then dip it into coconut flakes. Set aside. Shake all liquid ingredients with ice. Gently pour into rimmed glass.

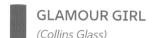

GLAMOUR GIRL
(Collins Glass)

Even if you don't land on the celebrity A List, "mommy" is the dream role for leading ladies waiting for baby's grand entrance. In the eyes of your little one, you'll always be the most beautiful woman in the world.

> 3 strawberries, diced
>
> 1 tablespoon torn basil
>
> ¾ ounce hibiscus Simple Syrup (recipe page 10)
>
> 4 ounces nonalcohlic rosé wine
>
> Splash of bitter lemon soda
>
> Additional whole strawberry

Muddle strawberries and basil in the bottom of a Collins glass. Add other ingredients and stir. Add ice and garnish with a strawberry on the rim of the glass.

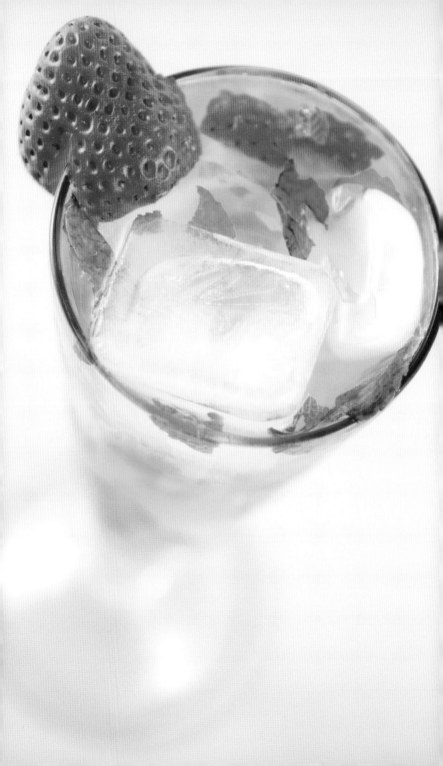

MOTHER TO THE KING
(Martini Glass)

Whether Queen Elizabeth II or Catherine Princess of Wales, our generation has seen at least two mothers of future monarchs in the British royal family. And despite breaking away from English rule more than two centuries ago, the royals remain an American pop culture obsession! Although we don't actually know what they prefer while pregnant, this Preggatini honors the queen in every mom-to-be.

>   4 ounces decaf Earl Grey tea
>
>   1 tablespoon orange marmalade
>
>   ¾ ounce grapefruit juice
>
>   ½ ounce lime juice
>
>   Orange twist
>
>   Shortbread cookie

Shake all ingredients with ice. Strain into a martini glass. Serve with the orange twist across the rim of the glass and shortbread cookie on the side.

Nightcaps

Okay, so maybe your rockstar stamina putters out around 8:00 p.m. nowadays. Slip on some comfy pajamas and indulge in your own nighttime ritual before baby baths and bedtime stories take over your evening hours. These Preggatinis are based on some favorite children's books and will help you relax at the end of the day too.

THE LAST APPLE, *THE GIVING TREE*
(Champagne Coupe)

Just when a mama feels she has nothing left to give, she'll dig deep to comfort her child. As you prepare for all the future holds, remember to take time to also nurture yourself in the busy months and years to come.

> 4 ounces spiced apple cider (cold or warm)
>
> 2 ounces ginger beer
>
> Red apple, sliced very thin

Pour cider and ginger beer into a champagne coupe. Slide the apple slices onto a drink pick, fan them out, and place on top of glass.

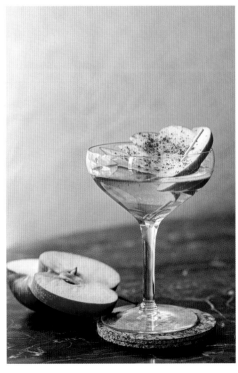

ASLAN'S SPELL, *THE CHRONICLES OF NARNIA*
(Collins Glass)

Aslan, the golden lion in this timeless book series, represents all that is good, fair, courageous, and generous in the world. Both protector and guide, he is a favorite character for children and adults alike. This drink will soothe and fortify you from the inside, out.

¾ ounce Simple Syrup (recipe page 10)

1 teaspoon powdered turmeric

4 to 5 ounces warm coconut milk

Marshmallows

Pour syrup into bottom of a Collins glass and stir in turmeric. Add warm coconut milk and stir. Treat yourself to some marshmallows on top!

MOONBEAMS AND SWEET DREAMS, *GOODNIGHT MOON*

(Wine Glass)

¾ ounce chamomile tea syrup (see page 10)

Powdered sugar

4 ounces coconut water

¼ ounce lemon juice

Rim the glass with powdered sugar and set aside. Shake coconut water, lemon juice, and chamomile tea simple syrup with ice. Gently strain into rimmed glass.

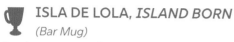

ISLA DE LOLA, *ISLAND BORN*
(Bar Mug)

Staying connected to their roots is important to every child's self-identity. This tale about Lola's desire to know where she came from is a sweet reflection of the very fabric that makes up America. This drink is inspired by Chocolate de Maní, a Dominican drink that is not actually made with chocolate, but with peanuts.

   ¼ cup roasted, unsalted peanuts

   1 cup cashew milk

   1 tablespoon sugar

   Pinch of ground cinnamon

   Pinch of nutmeg

   Pinch of ground clove

Blend all ingredients until completely smooth. Heat mixture in a small saucepan, stirring often, for about 5 minutes. Pour into mug and serve.

Themed Preggatini Party Menus for the Ultimate Baby Shower

As you may have gathered from (literally) everything in this book, I want to help you have fun while you're counting down the months to your baby's arrival. Well, what is more fun than your baby shower? Whether you are hanging out with a few close friends or throwing a big bash to remember, food and drinks are at the heart of any party. This section features three themed menus with delicious dishes and mocktails with moxie. Unless otherwise indicated, I've taught these dishes in The Liquid Muse cooking and cocktail classes, so I know they are winners!

Mexican Fiesta Preggatini Party

Hang a piñata, bust out some colorful platters, and turn up the tunes. These *delicioso* traditional Mexican recipes are bursting with flavor. Add some tortillas, rice, and maybe flan for dessert, and you've got a feast fit for a fiesta.

FRESH AND FRUITY
(Collins Glass)

Agua Fresca is a refreshing style drink all year round. It translates to "fresh water," and it really is that simple—water, fresh fruit, a bit of sugar. Below are just a couple of ideas. They can be made with any kind of fruit, so use what is in season near you and get creative.

PEACH AND GINGER

3 cups quartered peaches, skin on

2 tablespoons juiced ginger root

½ cup agave nectar (or to taste)

¼ cup lemon juice

4 cups water

Blend all together. Pour into a large pitcher. Stir before serving in ice-filled punch cups or Collins glasses.

WATERMELON AND MINT

3 cups cubed watermelon

¼ cup plucked mint leaves

½ raw sugar (or to taste)

¼ cup lime juice

4 cups water

Blend all together. Pour into a large pitcher. Stir before serving in ice-filled punch cups or Collins glasses.

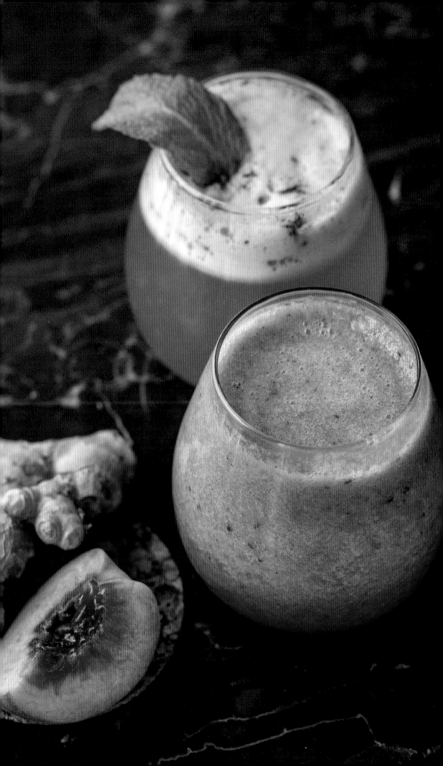

ROASTED SALSA

There are many ways to make salsa and, frankly, all of them are yummy. Personally, I love the rich flavor of roasted tomatoes and chilis with sweet pineapple. I like lots of garlic, too, but feel free to adjust this recipe to suit your taste buds.

> 1 tablespoon olive oil
>
> 3 large, ripe tomatoes, cut in half, seeds removed
>
> 4 green tomatoes (tomatillos)
>
> 3 jalapeño peppers, diced, seeds removed (could also use habanero or serrano peppers)
>
> ½ cup pineapple chunks (optional)
>
> 3 garlic cloves, diced
>
> ½ white onion, diced
>
> Pinch of salt (to taste)
>
> Juice from 1 lime
>
> 1 tablespoon diced cilantro (optional)
>
> Tortilla chips
>
> Carrot and/or jicama sticks

Heat oil on a griddle or in a large frying pan. Place tomatoes and peppers in the hot pan, cut side down. Let them cook until charred and blistering, then remove from heat. At this point, you could roast the pineapple, too, if desired. Grind or blend the garlic and onion with salt and lime juice, then add roasted tomatoes and chilis and pineapple. Hand mix or blend until desired smooth or chunky consistency. Serve with tortilla chips, carrot sticks, and sliced jicama.

OAXACAN ELOTE WITH AIOLI

In Mexico, it is common to find roasted corn cobs slathered in mayonnaise and sprinkled with crumbled white cotija cheese from street vendors. For parties, I prefer to serve this tasty combination as a side dish or in individual ramekins. It's easier to eat that way, but just as delicious.

1 cup olive oil

3 garlic cloves, peeled and cut in half

Salt, to taste

½ ounce lime juice

4 cups roasted corn kernels (roast cobs, or use frozen roasted corn)

¾ cup crumbled cotija cheese, divided in half

2 teaspoons red chili powder

Cilantro, chopped (optional)

Using a food processor or hand-held blender, mix a small amount of oil with garlic, salt, and lime juice. Slowly add more oil until mixture is a creamy and smooth aioli. Mix the aioli with corn and half the cotija cheese. Place in serving bowl then top with remaining cotija, red chili powder, and cilantro.

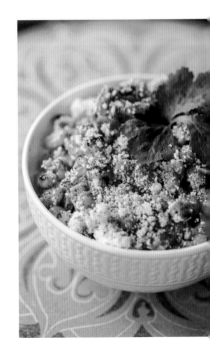

PEANUT MOLE WITH ROASTED CHICKEN THIGHS AND ACORN SQUASH

Although people outside of Mexico might equate mole with a savory dish made with chocolate, the word mole actually means sauce. I learned to make this peanut mole—containing no chocolate at all—in Oaxaca, and it is now one of my favorite sauces for white fish, fowl, and vegetarian meals.

TO PREPARE THE SQUASH AND CHICKEN:

Acorn squash, 1 for every 4 people

½ cup olive oil

Salt (to taste)

Chicken thighs, 1 per person

Cut acorn squash in half and remove seeds. Cut halves into quarters (resulting in eight pieces total). Brush each piece with olive oil and sprinkle with salt. Cook cut pieces in air fryer for 8 to 10 minutes, or roast at 425° Fahrenheit in oven for about 15 minutes.

Brush chicken thighs with oil and sprinkle with salt. Roast them in an air fryer for about 15 minutes or roast them with the vegetables in the oven for about 25 minutes or until skin is crispy and the liquid coming out of the thighs runs clear.

TO PREPARE THE PEANUT MOLE SAUCE:

½ cup olive oil, divided

1 yellow onion, diced

5 medium garlic cloves, diced

2 medium, ripe tomatoes

8 black peppercorns, crushed

1 teaspoon ground allspice

1 teaspoon ground cumin

2 tablespoons sesame seeds

2 whole cloves, crushed

1 cup shelled, unsalted peanuts

5 cups vegetable broth

4 ancho chiles

1 chipotle pepper (optional)

Salt to taste

Heat oil on low. Lightly sauté onions until softened, add garlic, tomatoes, crushed peppercorns, spices, and peanuts. Continue to stir until all are well mixed (about 5 minutes). Add ½ cup vegetable broth.

Raise heat to medium and slowly add remaining vegetable broth. Simmer for about 20 minutes, stirring often.

Let cool then ladle into blender. Blend for about 20 seconds, adding water if too thick. Mixture should be velvety but not watery. Once done, heat 2 teaspoons of oil in a saucepan and pour in the blended mixture. Simmer for about 15 minutes, adding a little water as needed. Spoon over the squash and chicken thighs.

Mediterranean Tapas Tasting

An escape to the crystal blue sea of southern Europe may not be on your horizon, but you can eat and drink as if you were there for your Preggatini Party. These tasty and easy menu ideas are sure to be on your dinner table for years to come. The mocktails in this chapter pull flavor from that sunny landscape. And the Mediterranean dip by celebrity chef Devin Alexander is a crowd pleaser for baby showers and parties, year-round. Add some almond biscotti or lemon tarts for sweets and your guests will be ooh-la-la-ing all afternoon.

 PREGGIE PROVENÇE
(Champagne Coupe)

Reminiscent of the tranquil hillsides of southern France, this Preggatini highlights fresh rosemary as well as lavender, for which La Provence is famous.

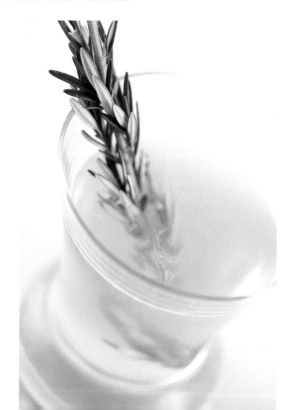

6 to 8 rosemary leaves

3 to 4 white grapes

¾ ounce lemon juice

1 ounce lavender Simple Syrup (recipe page 10)

3 ounces soda (If you can find lavender- or rosemary-flavored soda, that is ideal.)

1 lemon wheel

1 sprig rosemary

Muddle rosemary leaves and grapes in the bottom of a mixing glass or cocktail shaker. Add lemon juice and syrup, then shake well with ice. Strain into a champagne coupe. Top with soda, and garnish with a lemon wheel and a sprig of rosemary.

Extra Kick for Non-Preggie Pals: Add vodka, gin, or tequila.

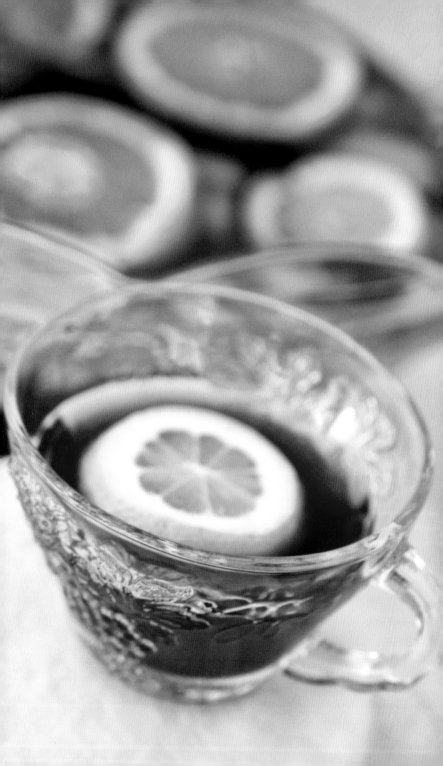

CITRUSY RED SANGRIA
(Wine Goblet)

This popular Iberian export can be made any time of the year, with red, white, or sparkling wine, and feature whichever fruits are in season. Mamas-to-be can enjoy them, too, when nonalcoholic wine is substituted.

- 1 orange, sliced with peel on
- 1 lemon, sliced with peel on
- 1 lime, sliced with peel on
- 2 cups tangerine (or orange) juice
- 1 cup nonalcoholic brandy or nonalcoholic rum
- ¾ cup hibiscus flower Simple Syrup (recipe page 10)
- ½ cup lemon juice
- 1 bottle nonalcoholic red wine

Mix all ingredients together, then cover and refrigerate at least 3 hours. Ladle into wine goblets or punch cups when ready to serve.

CRUISING THE MED CHARCUTERIE SKEWERS

Rather than the same old charcuterie board, offer these festive skewers, which are easy to make ahead of time and have a Mediterranean flair. Get creative with some of your favorite Mediterranean food. I offer three suggestions below, but you could add a Greek skewer with feta cheese, lemon chicken, and dolmas or a Moroccan one with lamb meatballs, dates, and roasted red pepper. Plan on serving 3 to 5 skewers per person.

SPANISH SKEWERS

Manchego cheese, cubed

Chorizo dried sausage, cut into ½-inch-thick pieces

Green olives, pitted

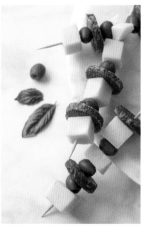

FRENCH SKEWERS

Brie or Camembert cheese, cubed

Cantaloupe or honeydew melon balls, 2 or 3 per skewer

Jambon de Bayonne (or prosciutto), 1 slice per melon ball

Black olives, pitted

ITALIAN SKEWERS

Mozzarella balls, 2 or 3 per skewer

Cherry tomatoes, 2 or 3 per skewer

Fresh basil leaves

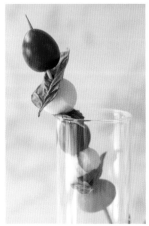

PAN CON TOMATE

When I lived in Spain, we made this with dinner almost every night. It's easy to prepare ahead of time and fun for guests to make themselves. Lunch tip: Toast your sandwich bread then follow the steps below. Fill with cold cuts, cheese, and veggies for a flavorful (and garlicky) sandwich.

> Toasted baguette slices (2 per person)
>
> Garlic cloves, peeled (1 per person)
>
> Ripe tomatoes, halved (1 half per person)
>
> Olive oil and salt, to taste

Rub the whole garlic cloves and the cut side of the tomatoes on the slices of toasted bread. Drizzle with olive oil and sprinkle with salt.

MEDITERRANEAN LAYER DIP WITH TOASTED PITA TRIANGLES

(Serves about 12)

This recipe is reprinted with permission from *The Most Decadent Diet Ever!* by my creative friend, celebrity chef Devin Alexander. She makes healthier options feel like off-limit treats.

1 cup garlic-flavored hummus

½ cup fat-free plain yogurt

¼ teaspoon ground cumin

½ teaspoon finely chopped fresh mint

1⅓ cups seeded and finely chopped cucumbers

1⅓ cups seeded and finely chopped Roma tomatoes

2 teaspoons finely chopped fresh parsley

1 teaspoon fresh lemon juice

1 teaspoon minced fresh garlic

Pinch of salt

¼ cup finely chopped red onion

3 ounces reduced-fat feta cheese, crumbled

2 tablespoons chopped Kalamata olives (about 8 olives)

6 (about 6½-inch-diameter) whole-wheat pita circles, lightly toasted and cut into wedges

"Life is too short for a bad meal . . . but even shorter if you eat too many bad-for-you meals. . . . There's nothing better than entertaining with healthier recipes and watching people enjoy food (and drinks!) that are actually good for them."

—Devin Alexander, *New York Times* bestselling *The Biggest Loser Cookbook*

Spoon the hummus into a 6-cup glass bowl. Use a spatula to spread it evenly to make one layer.

Mix the yogurt with the cumin and mint in a small bowl. Pour the yogurt mixture evenly over the hummus, and smooth it with the back of a spoon to form a second layer. Sprinkle the cucumbers evenly over the top.

Mix the tomatoes, parsley, lemon juice, garlic, and salt in a medium bowl. Sprinkle the tomato mixture over the cucumbers, followed by the onion, feta, then the olives.

Cover with plastic wrap and refrigerate for 1 to 6 hours. Serve with pita triangles for dipping.

Zen Chicks and Chill

If you would rather chill out than whoop it up, this Preggatini Party theme might be just your speed. There's an emphasis on calming ingredients and market-fresh presentation. The food and drink reflect this time of introspection and preparation (physical and mental) before the baby arrives. Some party ideas for this theme include hiring a massage therapist to give each guest a stress-relieving ten-minute shoulder rub, using the principles of feng shui to create an oasis in the baby's nursery, or starting a contest to see who can correctly predict baby's arrival and weight. You could gift the winner a gift certificate to the hippest yoga studio in town.

 ## YOGI-TEANI
(Wine Glass)

If you're the kind of person who needs her daily dose of Downward Dog and greets each day with a Sun Salutation, then this tea-based Preggatini will help you stay connected to your inner yogi. Deep breaths, sweet thoughts, tasty treats . . .

> 2 cups lemonade
>
> Approximately 14 raspberries
>
> 4 ounces Yogi Tea brand Woman's Mother to Be, room temperature
>
> 1 teaspoon raw brown sugar

Fill an ice cube tray with lemonade. Place 1 raspberry in each cube. Freeze.

When ice cubes are ready, pour tea and sugar into a mixing glass with regular ice and shake well. Strain into a wine glass. Drop in 2 or 3 raspberry-lemonade ice cubes.

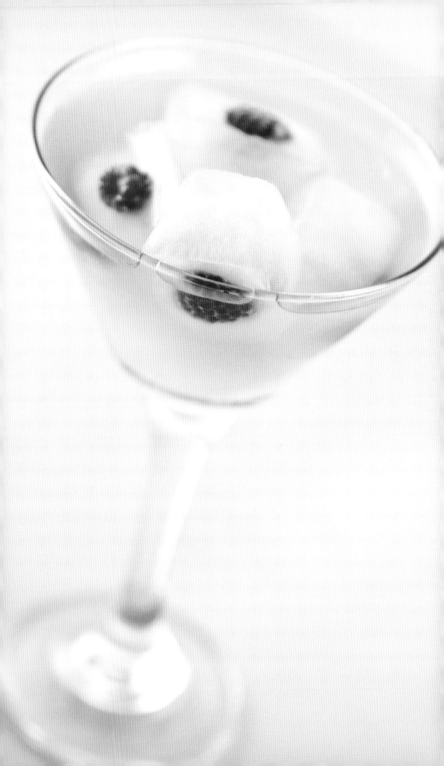

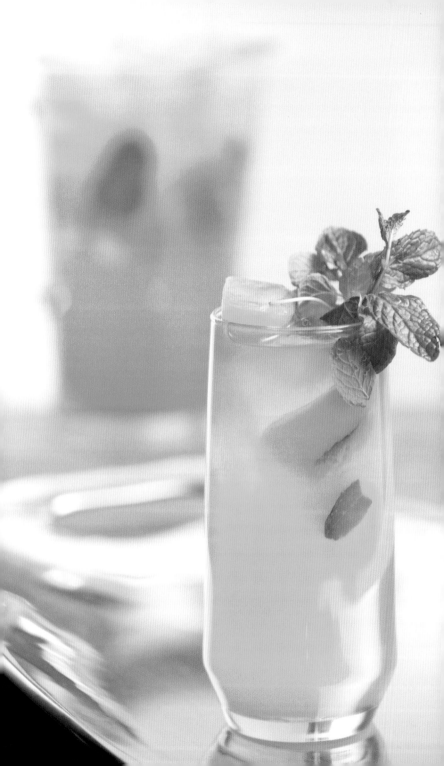

MINTY MANGO COOLER
(Collins Glass)

This simple punch tastes as good as it looks, and these swanky ice cubes make it look fancy. Fresh mint enhances both the flavor and the aroma.

> **2 cups mango juice mixed with 1 cup water, to make the ice cubes**
>
> **2 cups white grape juice**
>
> **3 cups mango juice**
>
> **2 cups bitter lemon soda**
>
> **3 trays mango ice cubes***
>
> **2 bunches fresh mint**

At least 3 hours before your party, pour the mango juice/water mixture into ice cube trays and put them in the freezer.

Pour white grape juice, mango nectar, and bitter lemon soda into a large pitcher or punch bowl. To serve, place 2 to 3 mango-mint ice cubes into a glass then add punch. Garnish each glass with a sprig of mint.

Extra Kick for Non-Preggie Pals: Add some vodka, gin, rum, or tequila.

LYCHEE SNOW CONE
(Martini Glass)

If you have a taste for exotic fruits, this delectable concoction will bang your gong. It can also be served as a liquid dessert for your zen celebration.

¼ ounce lychee syrup

2 ounces guava or passion fruit juice

2 ounces Greek yogurt, plain or vanilla

1 lychee fruit (canned)

Blend syrup, juice, and yogurt until mixed. Fill a martini glass with crushed ice, then pour in mixture. Top with lychee.

STEAMED BUNS

(Serves about 12)

In honor of the bun in your oven, these steamed buns will get everyone's attention. They are easy to prepare in a large quantity by scaling up the recipe. Stuff them with barbecue tofu, shredded chicken, pickled carrots and onions, spring onions, bean sprouts, and so on. Add some soy sauce and spicy red chili oil sauce on the side, and let guests help themselves.

> 2 teaspoons instant dry yeast
>
> 3 ounces lukewarm water
>
> 1¾ cups nondairy milk (soy works well for this recipe)
>
> 1 tablespoon sesame oil
>
> 2 teaspoons agave nectar
>
> 8 ounces gluten-free flour (rice flour is a great option)
>
> 1 teaspoon xanthan gum
>
> ½ teaspoon baking powder
>
> Pinch of salt

Activate yeast by mixing it well with the water. Add milk, oil, and agave nectar. Let stand until it starts to bubble (about 5 minutes).

Mix flour, xanthan gum, baking powder, and salt. Slowly pour the yeast mixture into the flour mixture until it is smooth. Continue to hand knead it on a floured surface or in a mixer with a dough hook. Add small amounts of water, if needed.

Let the dough rest about 15 minutes, then roll it out on a floured slab. Cut circles that are about 4 inches in diameter. Fold them in half and place them on parchment paper so they can rest at room temperature for a couple of hours. When ready to cook and fill the buns, steam them without filling for about 6 to 9 minutes. Add fillings and serve.

YELLOW TOMATO PARTY DIP WITH GRUYERE CHIPS

(Serves 6–8)

Early in my writing career, I wrote a monthly column called "Cooking with Michel" based on my walk-and-talks around Washington, DC, with celebrated chef, the late Michel Richard. In addition to his culinary musings, and cooking for luminaries at his legendary Georgetown eatery, Citronelle, the great restaurateur won the James Beard Foundation's 2007 Outstanding Chef Award and wrote the *Happy in the Kitchen* cookbook. Known for his palpable joie de vivre, he shared this sentiment along with the following recipe for this book.

DIP

1½ pounds large yellow tomatoes

1½ tablespoons finely minced shallots

1 garlic clove

1 teaspoon Dijon mustard

½ teaspoon soy sauce

¼ teaspoon granulated sugar

1 teaspoon chopped capers, drained

1 teaspoon minced chives

1 teaspoon extra virgin olive oil

Fine sea salt and freshly ground black pepper, to taste

Tabasco sauce, to taste

Preheat oven to 250°F.

Cut the cores from the tomatoes, then cut each tomato in half, lengthwise. Place cut side up on a parchment-lined baking sheet, and slowly roast for 3 hours.

Meanwhile, bring a small pan of water to a boil. Add the shallots and blanch quickly, just until tender. Drain in a fine-mesh sieve and run cold water over them to cool. Drain on a paper towel.

Remove tomatoes from oven. Discard the skins and scoop out the seedy centers. Chop the tomato flesh, place in the center of a cheesecloth, and wring out the excess liquid. Place the tomatoes in a medium bowl, add the shallots, and grate the garlic directly on top. Mix in the remaining ingredients and refrigerate until cold (at least 1 hour). Check the flavor again before serving, and adjust seasoning as needed.

GRUYERE CHIPS (GLUTEN FREE)

8 very thin slices of Gruyere (ask the deli to slice it for you)

2 tablespoons chopped chives

Preheat oven to 250°F.

Line a baking sheet with a nonstick baking mat and arrange cheese slices on it about 2 inches apart. Sprinkle with chopped chives. Bake about 15 minutes, until the cheese has melted and become golden brown. Remove from oven and let the chips firm up on the pan. When they are easy to remove, lift them with a spatula and place on paper towels or parchment paper to cool completely. Use the Gruyere chips to scoop the dip.

> "Friends are here to enjoy life with you. Present them with the food that you love. . . . Also, if you serve a special dish, print the recipe for your friends and let them take it home! Be creative, modern, have fun."
>
> —Michel Richard

CURRY YOGURT SALMON BITES

This light yet sophisticated appetizer from The Liquid Muse Events can easily translate to a main course by serving a filet of salmon with the luscious curry yogurt sauce. I created this bite-sized version, which can be easily nibbled from a buffet. Placed on a lettuce leaf, it is colorful, healthy, and gluten-free.

1 pound cubed salmon

3 tablespoons mustard oil

1 yellow onion, finely chopped

2 teaspoons red chili powder or cayenne pepper

2 teaspoons ground cardamom

1 teaspoon ground cinnamon

2 tablespoons grated fresh ginger

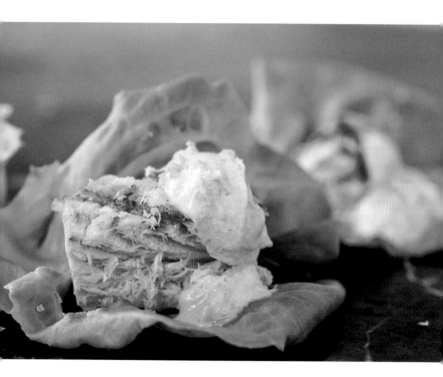

2 teaspoons ground turmeric

1 teaspoon salt

2 teaspoons ground cumin

1 tablespoon ground coriander

1 medium tomato, chopped

1½ cups water

½ cup Greek yogurt

1 bunch mint, finely chopped

Butter lettuce heads

Brush the salmon pieces with mustard oil, then air fry or bake them at 400° Fahrenheit until crispy. Set aside to let cool.

Heat remaining oil in a large skillet and add onion, chili powder (or pepper), cardamom, and cinnamon. Stir often until onions soften. Add ginger; mix well. Add remaining spices and mix well. Add tomatoes. Cook until tomatoes are soft, then add water, bring to a boil, reduce heat, and let simmer for about 8 minutes.

Let cool completely, then stir in the yogurt. Place a salmon cube on a butter lettuce leaf then drizzle with curry yogurt sauce.

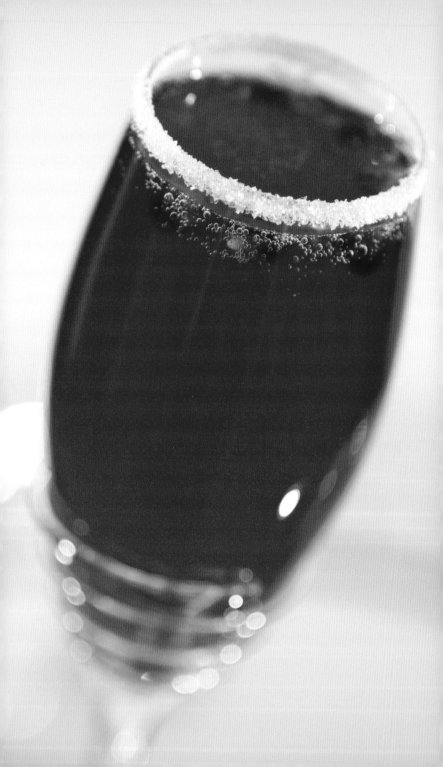

6

Holidays

No matter what time of year you're pregnant, you will encounter some holidays. But booze-free doesn't equal fun-free!

For those who normally (in a nonpregnant condition) would, oh, swig down a martini (or three) to deal with the pressure of hosting family gatherings 'round the turkey or planning a neighborhood Fourth of July picnic, don't sweat it. You will have a new form of "liquid courage" . . . your very own holiday-themed Preggatinis. Best of all, you can enlist well-intentioned but oh-so-meddlesome mother-in-law to make them for you. (Once she's having a ball shaking, muddling, and mixing, she'll have less opportunity to give you all those unsolicited mothering tips, and you'll wind up with a refreshing beverage. It's a win-win!)

One of the many great things about being pregnant around any holiday is indulging in extra helpings of all those special dishes people whip up at certain times of the year. Nurturing family and friends will ply you with seconds of Granny's coveted lasagna, your mom's nostalgic cheesecake, or your best friend's Christmas cookies—eating for two is fun, after all.

Even better, while everyone else is guzzling spiked eggnog, sipping holiday-themed martinis, or making slurry champagne toasts on New Year's Eve, you can find solace in knowing you will wake up without a hangover—or see pix you only kinda remember taking all over social media. In any case, before you know it, you will have more to celebrate than ever before—your baby!

NEW YEAR'S DAY: BABY NEW YEAR PUNCH
(Wine Glass)

While everyone else has sagging eyes and a pounding head, you'll be as fresh as a daisy on January 1. This twist on a Spanish kalimotxo is a great post-party brunch punch. For those who have indulged in a little too much the night before, the cola will help deliver sugar and caffeine (both of which help ease a hangover) and the nonalcoholic red wine will make it feel fun without further irritating their livers. In Spain, it is customary to eat twelve grapes when the clock chimes midnight, so freezing green and red grapes to use as ice cubes is a festive way to keep the drink chilled.

> **2 to 3 dozen red or green grapes**
>
> **2 cups cola (cane sugar Mexican Coca-Cola is ideal)**
>
> **2 cups nonalcoholic red wine**
>
> **2 to 3 dozen grape ice cubes**

Rinse grapes, space them apart on parchment paper, and freeze. I keep a supply of these in my freezer, but if you don't have any, be sure to allow 2 to 5 hours for them to freeze before you make your drinks!

Pour ingredients into a punch bowl. Add grape ice cubes to keep it chilled.

VALENTINE'S DAY: LOVE TRIANGLE
(Champagne Coupe or Flute)

You may have never considered celebrating Valentine's Day as a threesome, until now. As baby snuggles in your belly, picture next year's romantic soirée: you clutching a screaming, squirming bundle of joy in one arm as you hold your husband's hand across a candlelit table with the other—a whole new interpretation to the term *love triangle*!

¾ ounce Cantaloupe and Strawberry Shrub (recipe page 11)

4 ounces nonalcoholic sparkling wine

Heart-shaped lollipops

Pour shrub into champagne glass. Top with nonalcoholic sparkling wine. Garnish with a heart-shaped lollipop.

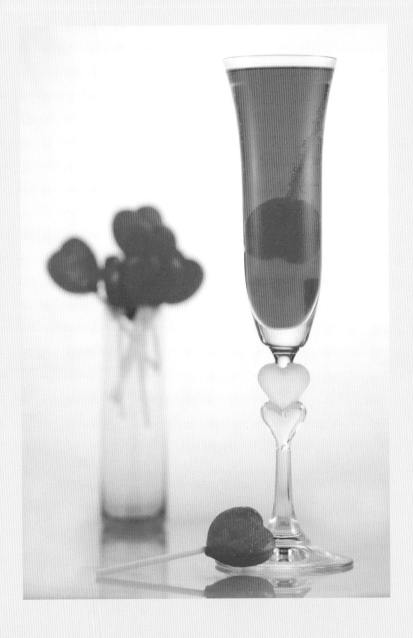

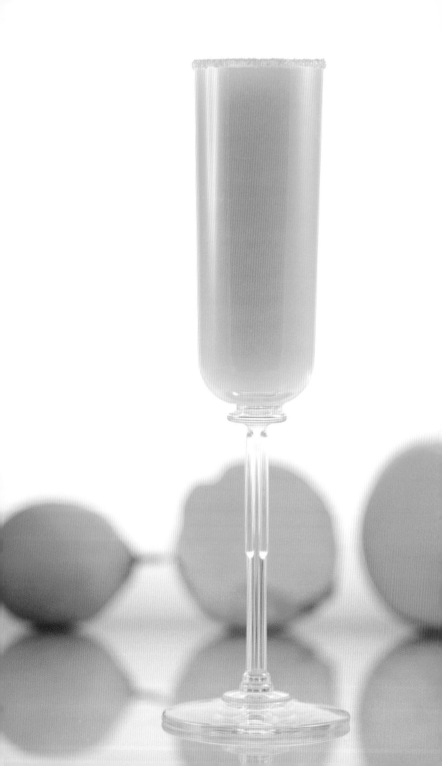

EASTER: SPARKLING CITRUS
(Champagne Coupe or Flute)

Do you love your mimosas at Easter brunch? This Preggatini is a more exciting version of what you're used to—even without the alcohol. Whether you are pregnant or simply abstaining from alcohol, this elegant sparkler complements everything from eggs Benedict to breakfast quiche.

Flavored cocktail rimming sugar

2 ounces pink grapefruit juice

2 ounces tangerine juice

Dash of grapefruit bitters (optional)

2 ounces blood orange soda

Rim a champagne glass with the sugar. Shake juices with ice, gently pour into champagne glass, then top with bitters (if desired) and blood orange soda.

MOTHER'S DAY: THE PERFECT PEAR
(Martini Glass)

This drink celebrates all things ripe, luscious, and curvy—including YOU! Whether you just found out you are pregnant or you're about to pop, raise a glass to yourself and your partner to acknowledge the perfect pair you make.

> **4 ounces pear juice**
>
> **¾ ounce lemon juice**
>
> **¾ ounce elderflower syrup**
>
> **Splash sparkling pear soda (or clear cream soda)**
>
> **Sprig of baby's breath**

Shake juices and syrup with ice. Strain into martini glass and top with soda. Use a tiny clothespin to attach a sprig of baby's breath flowers to the rim of the glass.

FATHER'S DAY: MY HONEYDEW
(Martini Glass)

"Honey do this, Honey do that . . ." will probably become common requests once the little one arrives and Mama needs an extra pair of hands. What better way to reward that awesome daddy for his partnerhship than by making him a refreshing cocktail you'll both enjoy?

  1 cup green tea

  1 cup sugar

  ½ cup honeydew melon chunks

  1½ ounces nonalcoholic rum

  ½ ounce lime juice

  Lime or lemon wedge

Warm the green tea and sugar until sugar melts to make a simple syrup. Set aside.

Muddle melon chunks, then add lime juice and ¾ ounce of green tea syrup. Shake well with ice. Strain into martini glass and sit a lime or lemon wedge on the rim.

Extra Kick for Non-Preggie Pals: Add 1½ ounces vodka, gin, or tequila and a splash of green melon liqueur.

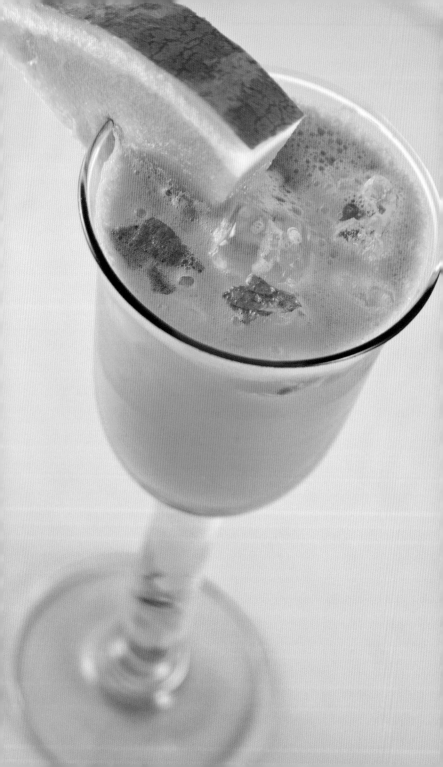

FOURTH OF JULY: WATERMELON COOLER
(Wine Goblet)

Punctuate an Independence Day picnic by sipping on America's favorite summertime fruit! This wonderfully refreshing Preggatini will be the envy of all your nonpregnant friends, so show them the "extra kick" directions below.

2 cups lemonade

6 to 8 mint leaves

½ ounce lime juice

6 ounces watermelon juice

1 tablespoon agave nectar

1 watermelon wedge

Fill ice cube tray with lemonade. Freeze

When lemonade cubes are frozen, muddle mint with lime juice. Add watermelon juice and agave nectar, shake with regular ice. Strain over lemonade ice cubes. Garnish with a watermelon wedge on the rim of the glass.

Extra Kick for Non-Preggie Pals: Add 1½ ounce of vodka, tequila, or rum.

> **TAKE ADVANTAGE OF SEASONAL FRUITS** to create your own Preggatinis using the recipe above as a guide. Muddle berries, chunks of pineapple or melon, peaches, figs, and so on with mint or basil or sage. Add a touch of sweetness and some citrus juice. Then shake it with ice. Any kind of fresh fruits make wonderful ingredients in both nonalcoholic and alcoholic cocktails.

LABOR DAY: GINGER BELLINI PUNCH
(Wine Glass)

Celebrating Labor Day (which is in September in the US) has a whole new meaning when you're preggers! The classic Bellini cocktail was created in Venice, Italy, in 1948. In this sparkling punch version, I added some raspberries for color and flavor. Let's make a special toast for working moms, too.

1 cup peach puree (or peach nectar)

Juice from 1 lemon

1 bottle nonalcoholic sparkling wine

½ cup fresh raspberries

Pour peach puree and lemon juice into a punch bowl. Stir. Slowly add nonalcoholic sparkling wine. Drop raspberries into the punch for a burst of color. Serve in wine glasses.

HALLOWEEN: GHOULISH GOBLET
(Wine Goblet)

The Espresso Martini has become very popular in recent years. This drink is reminiscent of that midnight delight and a fun offering for future Halloween parties.

4 ounces decaf coffee

2 ounces coconut cream

1 ounce blackberry-flavored syrup

½ teaspoon activated charcoal (Check with your doctor before using!)

Blackberries on a pick

Shake all ingredients with ice. Strain into ice-filled wine goblet. Lay blackberry pick on rim of glass.

Extra Kick for Non-Preggie Pals: Add 1½ ounce of vodka, tequila, rum, whiskey, or brandy.

THANKSGIVING: PUMPKIN PIE PREGGATINI
(Martini Glass)

If you love pumpkin pie, this Preggatini will remain a favorite long after the baby has arrived. Thick, creamy, and lip smackingly decadent, it's practically a dessert unto itself. (This is one of my personal favorites year-round!)

¾ ounce cinnamon syrup

3 tablespoons graham cracker crumbs (about 2 crackers)

1½ ounces nonalcoholic rum or nonalcoholic brandy

1½ ounces cream

1 heaping tablespoon sweetened condensed milk

1 heaping tablespoon canned pumpkin

Whipped cream

Pinch of ground cinnamon

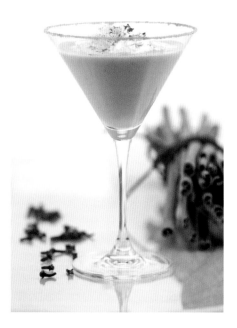

Wet rim of martini glass with cinnamon syrup, then dip it into the graham cracker crumbs and set aside. Vigorously shake other ingredients with ice. Slowly strain into rimmed martini glass. Top with a dollop of whipped cream and ground cinnamon.

HANUKKAH: BUBBLY BUBBALA
(Champagne Coupe)

Menorah candles aren't the only things that sparkle during the Festival of Lights! Whether you're spinning the dreidel, noshing on latkes, singing traditional songs, or exchanging gifts, this bubbly Preggatini will add a snazzy splash to the celebrations with its blue ice cube and nonalcoholic red wine.

> **2 cups blue pea flower tea**
>
> **3 ounces nonalcoholic red wine**
>
> **1 chocolate gold coin**

Fill ice cube tray with pea flower tea and freeze.

When cubes are ready, fill glass with nonalcoholic red wine. Garnish with one pea flower tea ice cube. Serve with chocolate gold coin.

CHRISTMAS: SPICE OF THE SEASON MULLED WINE

(Bar Mug)

Simmering spiced wine on the stove makes the whole house smell like the holiday season. With this nonalcoholic version, you can satisfy your taste buds when you take in that nostalgic smell (which may be amplified due to an enhanced sense of smell during pregnancy).

- 1 bottle nonalcoholic red wine
- 2 cups spiced apple cider
- 2 teaspoons almond extract
- 2 cinnamon sticks
- 1 whole orange, unpeeled, washed, and studded with cloves
- ¼ cup honey
- Orange slices or cinnamon sticks

Gently heat all ingredients. Stir until honey has dissolved. Serve in a bar mug. Or, if you live in a place where Christmas happens in the middle of summer, allow mixture to cool and serve this cold, over ice!

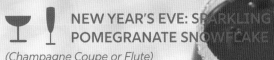

NEW YEAR'S EVE: SPARKLING POMEGRANATE SNOWFLAKE

(Champagne Coupe or Flute)

Top off a wonderful year with a special "champagne" cocktail. And just think: By this time next year, your baby will be celebrating with you!

- **2 tablespoons rimming sugar**
- **1 sugar cube**
- **Dash of orange bitters (optional)**
- **2 ounces pomegranate juice**
- **3 ounces nonalcoholic sparkling wine**
- **1 tablespoon pomegranate seeds**

Rim a champagne flute with sugar. Place sugar cube in the bottom of the flute, and, if desired, soak it with the bitters. Add pomegranate juice and nonalcoholic wine. Drop in pomegranate seeds.

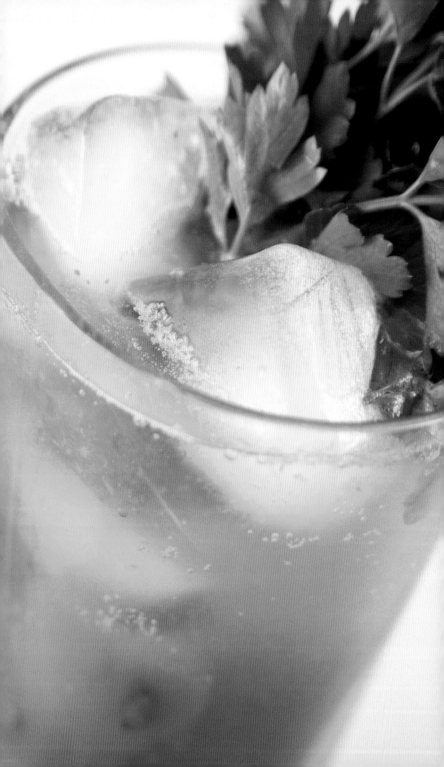

7

Breastfeeding and Beyond

Finally—the big moment is here. Yes, yes, the baby is wonderful, but what about getting the green light from your doctor to introduce small amounts of beer and wine back into everyday life?

Of course you should follow your intuition on this issue. I don't advocate boozing it up while breastfeeding by any stretch of the imagination. The beer, wine, and sparkling wine options offered here can also be made with nonalcoholic alternatives if you prefer to continue to abstain completely.

However, if you have medical approval and a desire to dip a toe into the pond of luscious low-alcohol libations, the recipes in this chapter will ease you back into imbibing.

Beer Cocktails

The words *beer* and *cocktail* may seem contradictory, but they play well together! Wonderful for summer barbecues or lounging by the lake, these cocktails dress up the average hot-dog-and-burger occasion.

 ## PANACHÉ
(Bar Mug)

Kissed with citrus and served ice-cold, this sunny refreshment is a favorite from the Mediterranean region.

>   **3 ounces beer, chilled**
>
>   **4 ounces bitter lemon soda**
>
>   **1 lemon wheel**

Pour chilled beer and bitter lemon soda into an ice-filled bar mug. Garnish with a lemon wheel. To avoid too much foam when pouring beer from a bottle or tap, tilt the glass slightly so that the beer runs down the side rather than hitting the bottom of the glass directly.

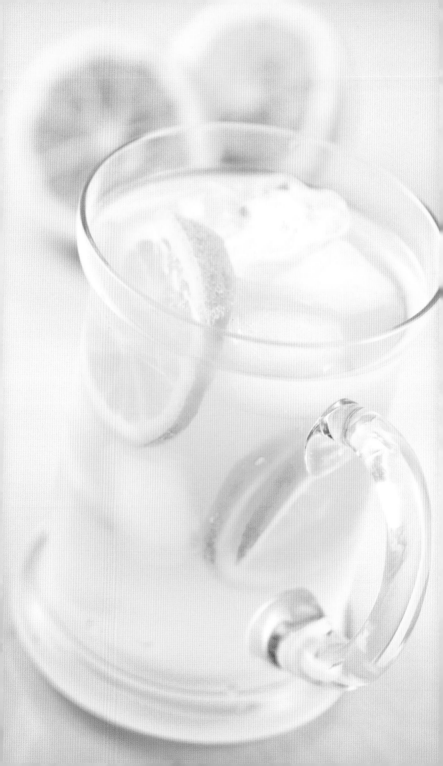

MEXICAN MICHELADA
(Bar Mug)

This brewed libation adds a splash of south-of-the-border flair to a backyard barbecue (great opportunity to show off the baby, of course), and brings a change of pace to taco night at home.

> 4 ounces Clamato juice
>
> ½ ounce lemon juice
>
> ½ ounce lime juice
>
> Dash of hot sauce
>
> Dash of Worcestershire or soy sauce
>
> 3 ounces pale Mexican beer
>
> Lime slice, celery stalk, and/or a leafy sprig of cilantro

Pour juices and condiments into a chilled bar mug or Collins glass. Add beer and stir. Add preferred garnishes.

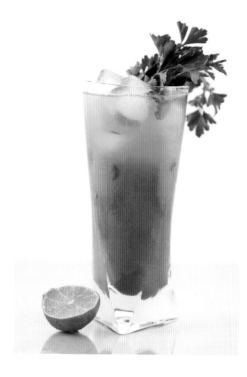

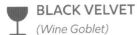

BLACK VELVET
(Wine Goblet)

Thick, creamy stout beer creates the bottom layer of this concoction, first dreamed up more than a century ago. Guinness is most commonly used, but you can experiment with any dark beer. Hard cider can also be substituted for champagne.

4 ounces stout beer

4 ounces champagne

Slowly pour beer, then champagne, into a wine goblet.

FACT OR FOLKLORE? Although it is widely believed that a small amount of beer is a natural remedy to help a nursing mom's milk flow, others recommend that babies drink no alcohol-laced breast milk. It is advisable to get your doctor's opinion before you conduct your own experiment.

Wine Cocktails

If you're a wine drinker, one of the biggest challenges during your pregnancy may have been giving up that playful Pinot Noir, forgoing your favorite bold California Zin, or turning down a glass of fancy French champagne. Now that you're ready to foray back into the vineyards, why not try a wine cocktail? Even winemakers who formerly cringed at the thought of anyone tinkering with vintages are reaching out to skilled mixologists.

FIRST CRUSH BLUSH
(Wine Glass)

Fruity and feminine, this wine spritzer gussies up a get-together with the girls.

> 3 strawberries, diced
>
> 1 ounce rose-infused Simple Syrup (recipe page 10)
>
> 3 ounces rosé wine
>
> Club soda
>
> 1 white rose

Muddle strawberries and rose-infused Simple Syrup in a mixing glass. Add ice and rosé wine then shake vigorously. Strain into a wine glass, and top with club soda. Garnish with a stemmed rose laid across the top of the glass.

"GREEN" AND WHITE SANGRIA
(Wine Glass)

This recipe is from The Liquid Muse "Sustainable Sips" organic cocktail class, and calls for biodynamic wine made from organic grapes grown with sustainable farming methods. I suggest Sauvignon Blanc because it has delightful hints of passion fruit, grapefruit, and kiwi.

1 cup organic peach nectar

2 bottles Sauvignon Blanc

2 cups chopped seasonal organic fruits (e.g., strawberries and peaches in summer, figs and pears in winter)

Mix peach nectar and wine. When ready to serve, spoon a tablespoon of fruit mixture into a wine glass. Fill with ice, then top with liquid. To prepare as a punch, place the fruit in a punch bowl, pour in peach nectar and wine. Chill for an hour, then let guests serve themselves with ice on the side so it doesn't water down the punch.

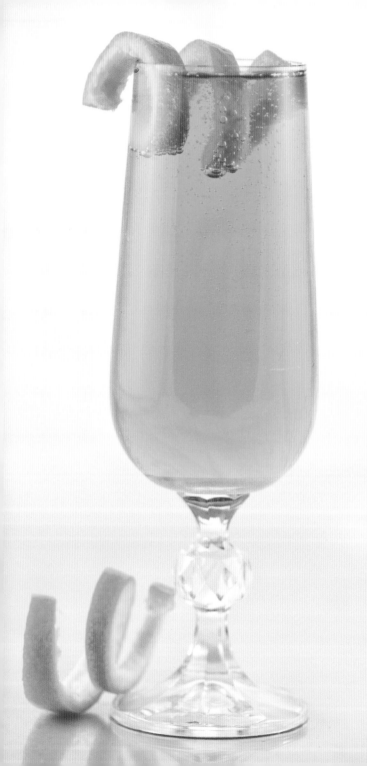

BISOUS DE PARIS CHAMPAGNE COCKTAIL
(Champagne Flute)

I love champagne with just about anything. When I combined it with port to make my version of a traditional champagne cocktail, I knew I'd found something I'd serve again and again. Now, you can too!

1 sugar cube

2 dashes of bitters

1½ ounces port

4 ounces champagne

1 orange peel twist

Douse a sugar cube with bitters and drop it into the bottom of a champagne flute. Add port and champagne. Garnish with an aromatic orange peel twist.

Low-Cal Preggatinis

Although the average baby weighs seven and a half pounds, women carry about four times that weight in fluids and tissue while the baby is growing. Although breastfeeding is nature's way of burning extra calories, keep in mind that one ounce of spirits has about seventy calories. If your fitness plan means kicking the booze for a bit longer, these Preggatinis will continue to satisfy you with only about fifty calories each.

HOT MAMA
(Martini Glass)

Hot peppers not only spice up your love life as natural aphrodisiacs, they also rev up your metabolism.

- 4 slices jalapeño, divided
- ½ ounce lime juice
- A few dashes of grapefruit bitters
- 3 ounces orange juice
- 2 ounces diet ginger ale

Muddle 1 jalapeño slice, lime juice, and bitters in the bottom of a mixing glass. Add orange juice and ice, then shake. Strain into a martini glass. Top with diet ginger ale. Garnish with the remaining jalapeño slices floating on the surface.

RANCH WATER PREGGATINI

(Collins Glass)

Grapefruits are so hailed for their fat-burning benefits that there is a whole diet fad created around them. This drink is by no means a meal replacement but rather an enhancement to any plan.

> 2 sections grapefruit, peeled
>
> Basil, about 8 leaves
>
> ½ ounce lemon juice
>
> 1½ ounces grapefruit juice
>
> 3 ounces diet tonic water

Muddle grapefruit, basil, and lemon juice in the bottom of a Collins glass. Add ice and grapefruit juice. Top with tonic water.

COSMOMPOLITAN COOLER
(Collins Glass)

Pour this Preggatini into a Martini glass and you won't miss a thing—except a little buzz—at the next sparkling soirée.

2 ounces cranberry juice

1 ounce lime juice

Dash of orange bitters

4 ounces citrus-flavored sparkling water

Lime wedge

Fill a Collins glass with ice and pour in all liquid ingredients. Stir with a bar spoon. Slide lime wedge onto the rim of the glass.

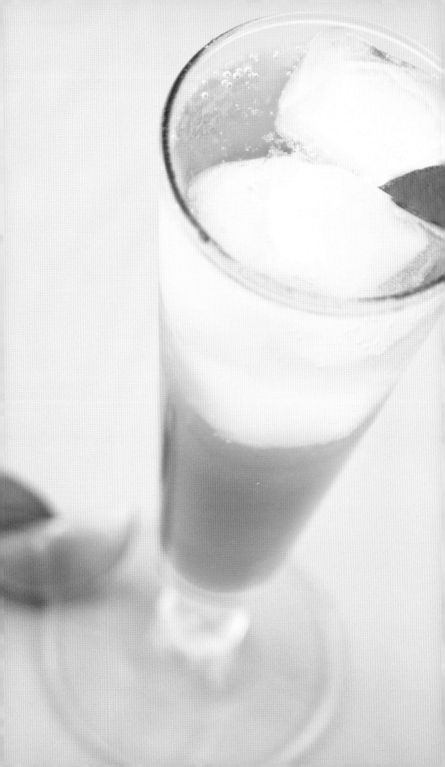

Index

About the Author

Natalie Bovis is an award-winning mixologist, event producer, author, and founder of The Liquid Muse. She is the co-founder of OM Chocolate Liqueur and New Mexico Cocktail Week. She produces creativity, culinary, and yoga retreats, the Cocktails & Culture festival, and special dinners for clients, including the James Beard Foundation. Natalie volunteers with animal rescues, and part of her personal mission is raising money for animal advocacy groups. She teaches cocktail and cooking classes and has shaken up cocktails and mocktails on television shows across the United States. Natalie is the American-born daughter of an English mum and French dad and has lived and worked in Santa Fe, Los Angeles, Paris, Washington, DC, and the Costa Brava in Spain. Her passions include protecting wildlife and the environment, traveling, cooking, hiking, and writing articles, poetry, fiction, and nonfiction. Her other cocktail books include *Edible Cocktails: From Garden to Glass; Drinking with My Dog: The Canine Lover's Cocktail Book;* and *Cocktails with My Cat: Tasty Tipples for Feline Fanatics.* Share more cocktail fun with Natalie at TheLiquidMuse.com and @theliquidmuse on the socials.